Virtual Clinical Excursions—Pediatrics

Virtual Clinical Excursions—Pediatrics

software developed by

Wolfsong Informatics, LLC
Tucson, Arizona

ELSEVIER

ELSEVIER

3251 Riverport Lane
Maryland Heights, Missouri 63043

VIRTUAL CLINICAL EXCURSIONS—PEDIATRICS
Copyright © 2017, Elsevier Inc. All rights reserved.

ISBN: 978-0-323-49814-2

Notice

Knowledge and best practice in this field are constantly changing. As new research and experience broaden our understanding, changes in research methods, professional practices, or medical treatment may become necessary.

Practitioners and researchers must always rely on their own experience and knowledge in evaluating and using any information, methods, compounds, or experiments described herein. In using such information or methods they should be mindful of their own safety and the safety of others, including parties for whom they have a professional responsibility.

With respect to any drug or pharmaceutical products identified, readers are advised to check the most current information provided (i) on procedures featured or (ii) by the manufacturer of each product to be administered, to verify the recommended dose or formula, the method and duration of administration, and contraindications. It is the responsibility of practitioners, relying on their own experience and knowledge of their patients, to make diagnoses, to determine dosages and the best treatment for each individual patient, and to take all appropriate safety precautions.

To the fullest extent of the law, neither the Publisher nor the authors, contributors, or editors, assume any liability for any injury and/or damage to persons or property as a matter of products liability, negligence or otherwise, or from any use or operation of any methods, products, instructions, or ideas contained in the material herein.

ISBN: 978-0-323-49814-2

Printed in the United States of America

Last digit is the print number: 9   8   7   6   5   4   3   2   1

Table of Contents
Virtual Clinical Excursions Workbook

GETTING SET UP WITH VCE ONLINE

The product you have purchased is part of the Evolve Learning System. Please read the following information thoroughly to get started.

■ HOW TO ACCESS YOUR VCE RESOURCES ON EVOLVE

There are two ways to access your VCE Resources on Evolve:

1. If your instructor has enrolled you in your VCE Evolve Resources, you will receive an email with your registration details.

2. If your instructor has asked you to self-enroll in your VCE Evolve Resources, he or she will provide you with your Course ID (for example, 1479_jdoe73_0001). You will then need to follow the instructions at https://evolve.elsevier.com/cs/studentEnroll.html.

■ HOW TO ACCESS THE ONLINE VIRTUAL HOSPITAL

The online virtual hospital is available through the Evolve VCE Resources. There is no software to download or install: the online virtual hospital runs within your Internet browser, using a pop-up window.

■ TECHNICAL REQUIREMENTS

- Broadband connection (DSL or cable)
- 1024 x 768 screen resolution
- Mozilla Firefox 18.0, Internet Explorer 9.0, Google Chrome, or Safari 5 (or higher)
  Note: Pop-up blocking software/settings must be disabled.
- Adobe Acrobat Reader
- Additional technical requirements available at http://evolvesupport.elsevier.com

■ HOW TO ACCESS THE WORKBOOK

There are two ways to access the workbook portion of *Virtual Clinical Excursions:*

1. Print workbook
2. An electronic version of the workbook, available within the VCE Evolve Resources

■ TECHNICAL SUPPORT

Technical support for *Virtual Clinical Excursions* is available by visiting the Technical Support Center at http://evolvesupport.elsevier.com or by calling 1-800-222-9570 inside the United States and Canada.

Trademarks: Windows® and Macintosh® are registered trademarks.

A QUICK TOUR

Welcome to *Virtual Clinical Excursions—Pediatrics*, a virtual hospital setting in which you can work with multiple complex patient simulations and also learn to access and evaluate the information resources that are essential for high-quality patient care. The virtual hospital, Pacific View Regional Hospital, has realistic architecture and access to patient rooms, a Nurses' Station, and a Medication Room.

■ BEFORE YOU START

Make sure you have your textbook nearby when you use *Virtual Clinical Excursions*. You will want to consult topic areas in your textbook frequently while working with the virtual hospital and workbook.

■ HOW TO SIGN IN

- Enter your name on the Student Nurse identification badge.
- Now choose one of the four periods of care in which to work. In Periods of Care 1 through 3, you can actively engage in patient assessment, entry of data in the electronic patient record (EPR), and medication administration. Period of Care 4 presents the day in review. Highlight and click the appropriate period of care. (For this quick tour, choose **Period of Care 1: 0730-0815**.)
- This takes you to the Patient List screen (see the *How to Select a Patient* section below). Only the patients on the Pediatrics Floor are available. Note that the virtual time is provided in the box at the lower left corner of the screen (0730, since we chose Period of Care 1).

Note: If you choose to work during Period of Care 4: 1900-2000, the Patient List screen is skipped since you are not able to visit patients or administer medications during the shift. Instead, you are taken directly to the Nurses' Station, where the records of all the patients on the floor are available for your review.

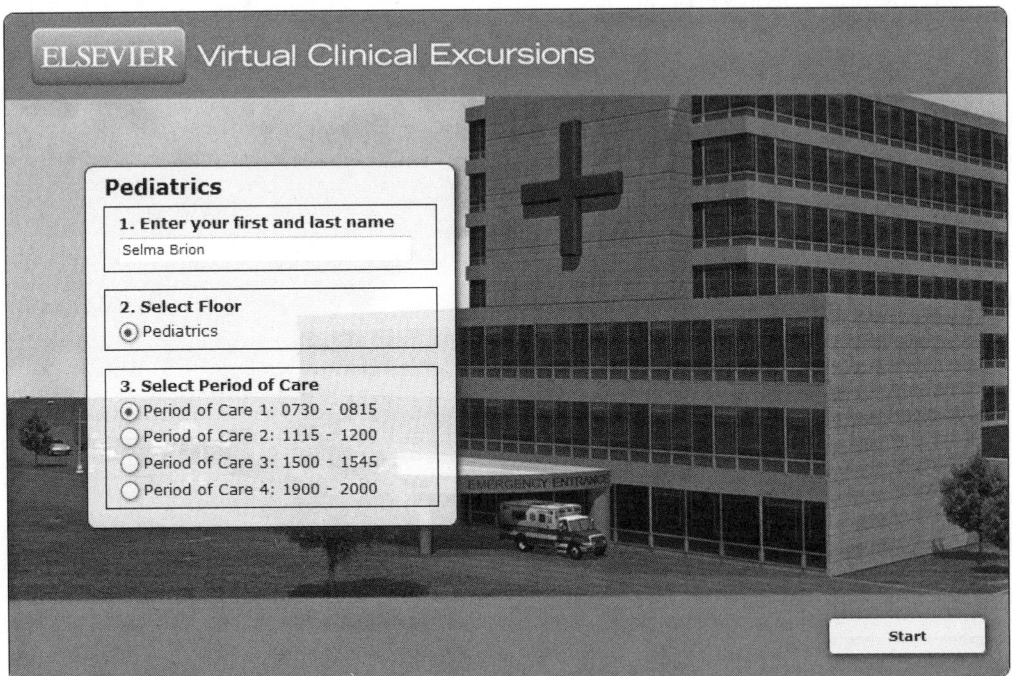

■ PATIENT LIST

PEDIATRICS UNIT

George Gonzalez (Room 301)
Diabetic ketoacidosis—An 11-year-old Hispanic male admitted for stabilization of blood glucose level and diabetic re-education associated with his diagnosis of type 1 diabetes mellitus. This patient's poor compliance with insulin therapy and dietary regime have resulted in frequent and repeated hospital admissions for diabetic ketoacidosis.

Tommy Douglas (Room 302)
Traumatic brain injury—A 6-year-old Caucasian male transferred from the Pediatric Intensive Care Unit in preparation for organ donation. This patient is status post ventriculostomy with negative intracerebral blood flow and requires extensive hemodynamic monitoring and support, along with compassionate family care.

Carrie Richards (Room 303)
Bronchiolitis—A 3½-month-old African-American female admitted with respiratory distress due to respiratory syncytial virus, along with dehydration and a poor nutritional status. Parent education and support are among her primary needs.

Stephanie Brown (Room 304)
Meningitis—A 3-year-old African-American female with a history of spastic cerebral palsy admitted for intravenous antibiotic therapy, neurologic monitoring, and support for a diagnosis of acute meningitis. Maintenance of physical and occupational programs addressing her mobility limitations complicate her acute care stay.

Tiffany Sheldon (Room 305)
Anorexia nervosa—A 14-year-old Caucasian female admitted for dehydration, electrolyte imbalance, and malnutrition following a syncope episode at home. This patient has a history of eating disorders, which have resulted in multiple hospital admissions and strained family dynamics between mother and daughter.

■ HOW TO SELECT A PATIENT

- You can choose one or more patients to work with from the Patient List by checking the box to the left of the patient name(s). For this quick tour, select Stephanie Brown. (In order to receive a scorecard for a patient, the patient must be selected before proceeding to the Nurses' Station.)
- Click on **Get Report** to the right of the medical records number (MRN) to view a summary of the patient's care during the 12-hour period before your arrival on the unit.
- After reviewing the report, click on **Go to Nurses' Station** in the right lower corner to begin your care. (*Note:* If you have been assigned to care for multiple patients, you can click on **Return to Patient List** to select and review the report for each additional patient before going to the Nurses' Station.)

Note: Even though the Patient List is initially skipped when you sign in to work for Period of Care 4, you can still access this screen if you wish to review the shift report for any of the patients. To do so, simply click on **Patient List** near the top left corner of the Nurses' Station (or click on the clipboard to the left of the Kardex). Then click on **Get Report** for the patient(s) whose care you are reviewing. This may be done during any period of care.

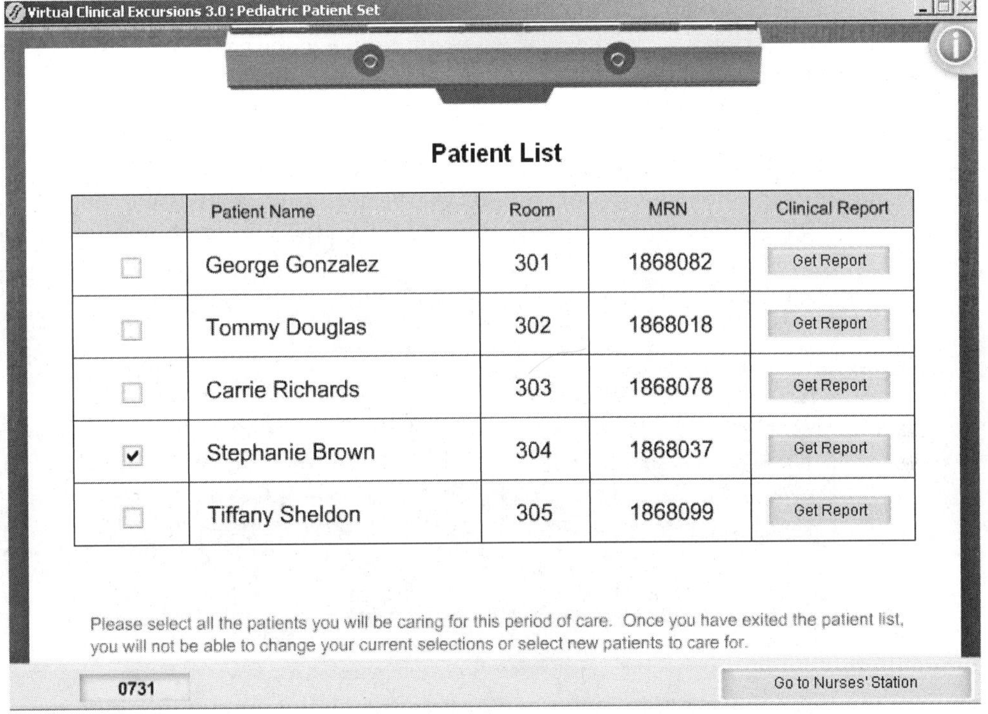

	Patient Name	Room	MRN	Clinical Report
☐	George Gonzalez	301	1868082	Get Report
☐	Tommy Douglas	302	1868018	Get Report
☐	Carrie Richards	303	1868078	Get Report
☑	Stephanie Brown	304	1868037	Get Report
☐	Tiffany Sheldon	305	1868099	Get Report

■ HOW TO FIND A PATIENT'S RECORDS

NURSES' STATION

Within the Nurses' Station, you will see:

1. A clipboard that contains the patient list for that floor.
2. A chart rack with patient charts labeled by room number, a notebook labeled Kardex, and a notebook labeled MAR (Medication Administration Record).
3. A desktop computer with access to the Electronic Patient Record (EPR).
4. A tool bar across the top of the screen that can also be used to access the Patient List, EPR, Chart, MAR, and Kardex. This tool bar is also accessible from each patient's room.
5. A Drug Guide containing information about the medications you are able to administer to your patients.
6. A Laboratory Guide containing normal value ranges for all laboratory tests you may come across in the virtual patient hospital.
7. A tool bar across the bottom of the screen that can be used to access the Floor Map, patient rooms, Medication Room, and Drug Guide.

As you run your cursor over an item, it will be highlighted. To select, simply click on the item. As you use these resources, you will always be able to return to the Nurses' Station by clicking on the **Return to Nurses' Station** bar located in the right lower corner of your screen.

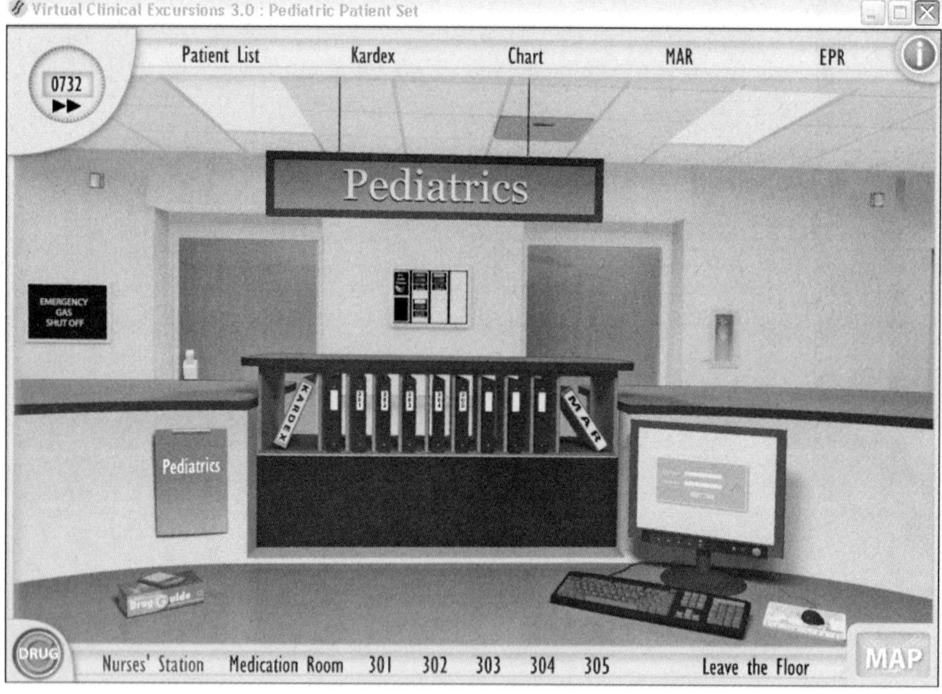

MEDICATION ADMINISTRATION RECORD (MAR)

The MAR icon located on the tool bar at the top of your screen accesses current 24-hour medications for each patient. Click on the icon and the MAR will open. (*Note:* You can also access the MAR by clicking on the MAR notebook on the far right side of the book rack in the center of the screen.) Within the MAR, tabs on the right side of the screen allow you to select patients by room number. Be careful to make sure you select the correct tab number for *your* patient rather than simply reading the first record that appears after the MAR opens. Each MAR sheet lists the following:

- Medications
- Route and dosage of each medication
- Times of administration of each medication

Note: The MAR changes each day. Expired MARs are stored in the patients' charts.

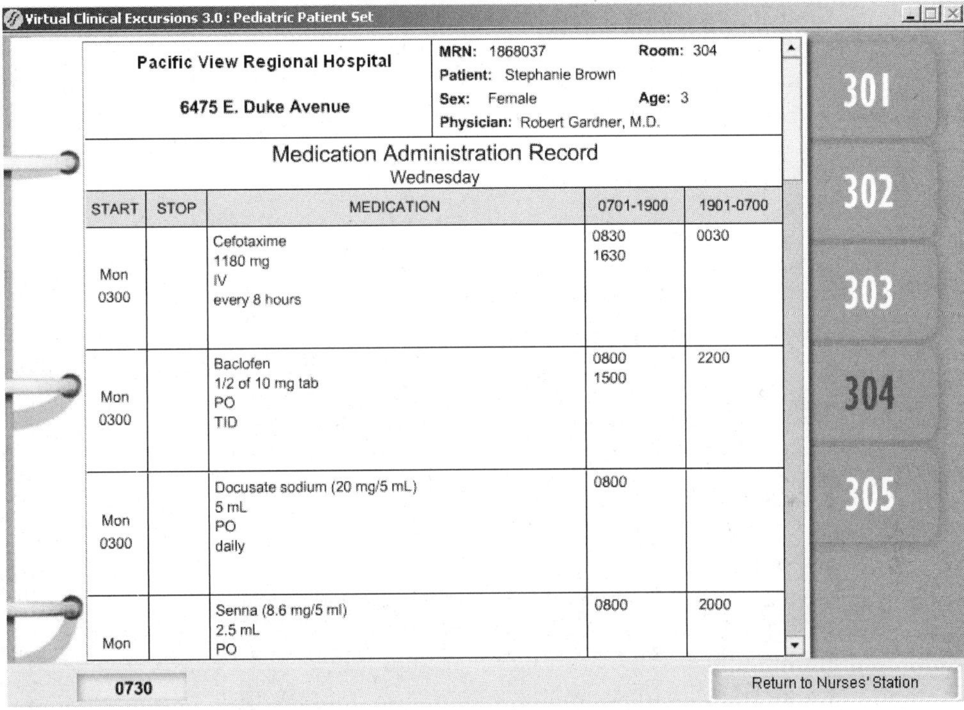

START	STOP	MEDICATION	0701-1900	1901-0700
Mon 0300		Cefotaxime 1180 mg IV every 8 hours	0830 1630	0030
Mon 0300		Baclofen 1/2 of 10 mg tab PO TID	0800 1500	2200
Mon 0300		Docusate sodium (20 mg/5 mL) 5 mL PO daily	0800	
Mon		Senna (8.6 mg/5 ml) 2.5 mL PO	0800	2000

CHARTS

To access patient charts, either click on the **Chart** icon at the top of your screen or anywhere within the chart rack in the center of the Nurses' Station screen. When the close-up view appears, the individual charts are labeled by room number. To open a chart, click on the room number of the patient whose chart you wish to review. The patient's name and allergies will appear on the left side of the screen, along with a list of tabs on the right side of the screen, allowing you to view the following data:

- Allergies
- Physician's Orders
- Physician's Notes
- Nurse's Notes
- Laboratory Reports
- Diagnostic Reports
- Surgical Reports
- Consultations

- Patient Education
- History and Physical
- Nursing Admission
- Expired MARs
- Consents
- Mental Health
- Admissions
- Emergency Department

Information appears in real time. The entries are in reverse chronologic order, so use the down arrow at the right side of each chart page to scroll down to view previous entries. Flip from tab to tab to view multiple data fields or click on **Return to Nurses' Station** in the lower right corner of the screen to exit the chart.

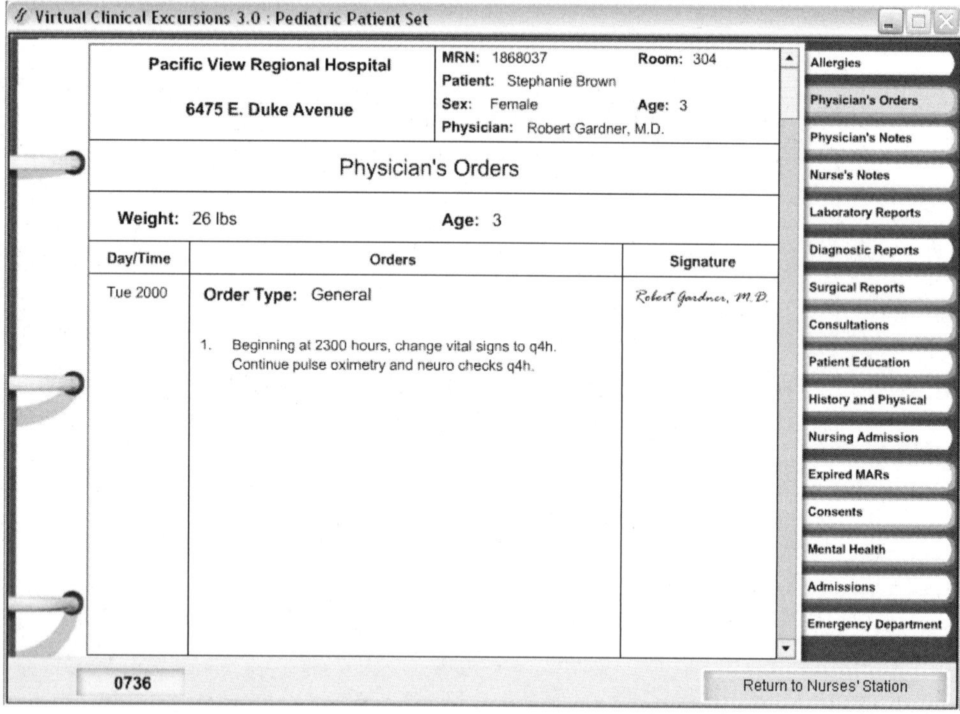

ELECTRONIC PATIENT RECORD (EPR)

The EPR can be accessed from the computer in the Nurses' Station or from the EPR icon located in the tool bar at the top of your screen. To access a patient's EPR:

- Click on either the computer screen or the **EPR** icon.
- Your username and password are automatically filled in.
- Click on **Login** to enter the EPR.
- *Note:* Like the MAR, the EPR is arranged numerically. Thus when you enter, you are initially shown the records of the patient in the lowest room number on the floor. To view the correct data for *your* patient, remember to select the correct room number, using the drop-down menu for the Patient field at the top left corner of the screen.

The EPR used in Pacific View Regional Hospital represents a composite of commercial versions being used in hospitals. You can access the EPR:

- to review existing data for a patient (by room number).
- to enter data you collect while working with a patient.

The EPR is updated daily, so no matter what day or part of a shift you are working, there will be a current EPR with the patient's data from the past days of the current hospital stay. This type of simulated EPR allows you to examine how data for different attributes have changed over time, as well as to examine data for all of a patient's attributes at a particular time. The EPR is fully functional (as it is in a real-life hospital). You can enter such data as blood pressure, breath sounds, and certain treatments. The EPR will not, however, allow you to enter data for a previous time period. Use the arrows at the bottom of the screen to move forward and backward in time.

Patient Room: 304	**Category:** Vital Signs			**Electronic Patient Records**
Name: Stephanie Brown	Wed 0300	Wed 0700	Wed 0730	Code Meanings
PAIN: LOCATION				
PAIN: RATING	0	0		
PAIN: CHARACTERISTICS				
PAIN: VOCAL CUES				
PAIN: FACIAL CUES				
PAIN: BODILY CUES				
PAIN: SYSTEM CUES				
PAIN: FUNCTIONAL EFFECTS				
PAIN: PREDISPOSING FACTORS				
PAIN: RELIEVING FACTORS				
PCA				
TEMPERATURE (F)	98.6	97.6		
TEMPERATURE (C)				
MODE OF MEASUREMENT	Ty	Ty		
SYSTOLIC PRESSURE	80	92		
DIASTOLIC PRESSURE	42	50		
BP MODE OF MEASUREMENT	NIBP	NIBP		
HEART RATE	98	92		
RESPIRATORY RATE	22	20		
SpO2 (%)	100	99		
BLOOD GLUCOSE				
WEIGHT	20	11.82		
HEIGHT				

0731

Return to Nurses' Station

At the top of the EPR screen, you can choose patients by their room numbers. In addition, you have access to 17 different categories of patient data. To change patients or data categories, click the down arrow to the right of the room number or category.

The categories of patient data in the EPR are as follows:

- Vital Signs
- Respiratory
- Cardiovascular
- Neurologic
- Gastrointestinal
- Excretory
- Musculoskeletal
- Integumentary
- Reproductive
- Psychosocial
- Wounds and Drains
- Activity
- Hygiene and Comfort
- Safety
- Nutrition
- IV
- Intake and Output

Remember, each hospital selects its own codes. The codes used in the EPR at Pacific View Regional Hospital may be different from ones you have seen in your clinical rotations. Take some time to acquaint yourself with the codes. Within the Vital Signs category, click on any item in the left column (e.g., Pain: Characteristics). In the far-right column, you will see a list of code meanings for the possible findings and/or descriptors for that assessment area.

You will use the codes to record the data you collect as you work with patients. Click on the box in the last time column to the right of any item and wait for the code meanings applicable to that entry to appear. Select the appropriate code to describe your assessment findings and type it in the box. (*Note:* If no cursor appears within the box, click on the box again until the blue shading disappears and the blinking cursor appears.) Once the data are typed in this box, they are entered into the patient's record for this period of care only.

To leave the EPR, click on **Exit EPR** in the bottom right corner of the screen.

■ VISITING A PATIENT

From the Nurses' Station, click on the room number of the patient you wish to visit (in the tool bar at the bottom of your screen). Once you are inside the room, you will see a still photo of your patient in the top left corner. To verify that this is the correct patient, click on the **Check Armband** icon to the right of the photo. The patient's identification data will appear. If you click on **Check Allergies** (the next icon to the right), a list of the patient's allergies (if any) will replace the photo.

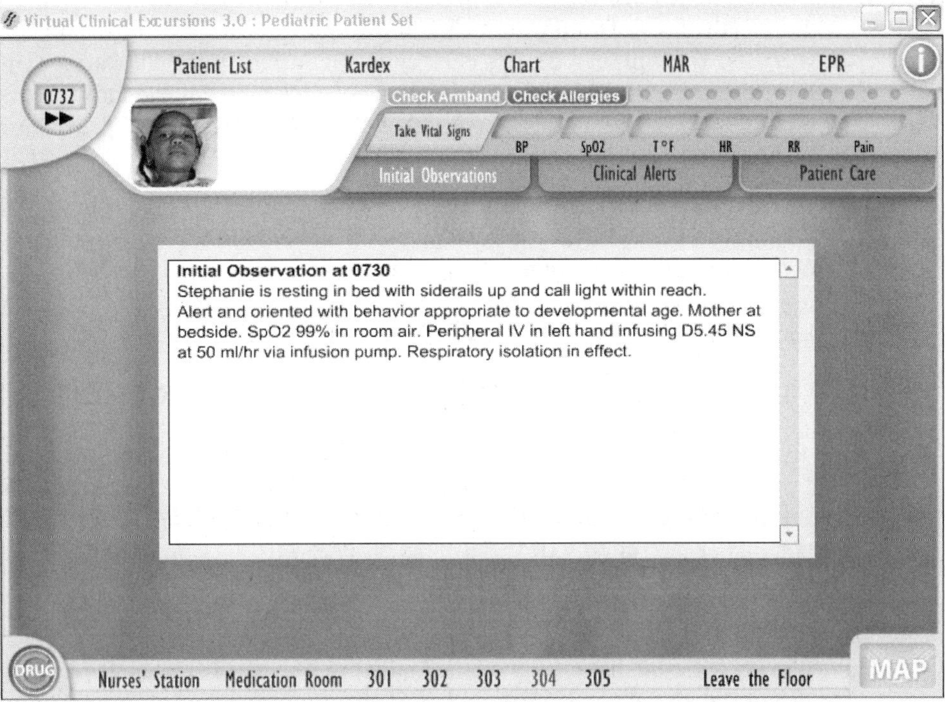

Also located in the patient's room are multiple icons you can use to assess the patient or the patient's medications. A virtual clock is provided in the upper left corner of the room to monitor your progress in real time. (*Note:* The fast-forward icon within the virtual clock will advance the time by 2-minute intervals when clicked.)

- The tool bar across the top of the screen allows you to check the **Patient List**, access the **EPR** to check or enter data, and view the patient's **Chart**, **MAR**, or **Kardex**.

- The **Take Vital Signs** icon allows you to measure the patient's up-to-the-minute blood pressure, oxygen saturation, temperature, heart rate, respiratory rate, and pain level.

- Each time you enter a patient's room, you are given an Initial Observation report to review (in the text box under the patient's photo). These notes are provided to give you a "look" at the patient as if you had just stepped into the room. You can also click on the **Initial Observations** icon to return to this box from other views within the patient's room. To the right of this icon is **Clinical Alerts**, a resource that allows you to make decisions about priority medication interventions based on emerging data collected in real time. Check this screen throughout your period of care to avoid missing critical information related to recently ordered or STAT medications.

- Clicking on **Patient Care** opens up three specific learning environments within the patient room: **Physical Assessment**, **Nurse-Client Interactions**, and **Medication Administration**.

- To perform a **Physical Assessment**, choose a body area (such as **Head & Neck**) from the column of yellow buttons. This activates a list of system subcategories for that body area (e.g., see **Sensory**, **Neurologic**, etc. in the green boxes). After you select the system you wish to evaluate, a brief description of the assessment findings will appear in a box to the right. A still photo provides a "snapshot" of how an assessment of this area might be done or what the finding might look like. For every body area, you can also click on **Equipment** on the right side of the screen.

- To the right of the Physical Assessment icon is **Nurse-Client Interactions**. Clicking on this icon will reveal the times and titles of any videos available for viewing. (*Note:* If the video you wish to see is not listed, this means you have not yet reached the correct virtual time to view that video. Check the virtual clock; you may return to access the video once its designated time has occurred—as long as you do so within the same period of care. Or you can click on the fast-forward icon within the virtual clock to advance the time by 2-minute intervals. You will then need to click again on **Patient Care** and **Nurse-Client Interactions** to refresh the screen.) To view a listed video, click on the white arrow to the right of the video title. Use the control buttons below the video to start, stop, pause, rewind, or fast-forward the action or to mute the sound.

- **Medication Administration** is the pathway that allows you to review and administer medications to a patient after you have prepared them in the Medication Room. This process is also addressed further in the *How to Prepare Medications* section below and in *Medications* in **A Detailed Tour**. For additional hands-on practice, see *Reducing Medication Errors* below **A Quick Tour** and **A Detailed Tour** in your resources.

■ HOW TO QUIT, CHANGE PATIENTS, OR CHANGE PERIODS OF CARE

How to Quit: From most screens, you may click the **Leave the Floor** icon on the bottom tool bar to the right of the patient room numbers. (*Note:* From some screens, you will first need to click an **Exit** button or **Return to Nurses' Station** before clicking **Leave the Floor**.) When the Floor Menu appears, click **Exit** to leave the program.

How to Change Patients or Periods of Care: To change patients, simply click on the new patient's room number. (You cannot receive a scorecard for a new patient, however, unless you have already selected that patient on the Patient List screen.) To change to a new period of care or to restart the virtual clock, click on **Leave the Floor** and then on **Restart the Program**.

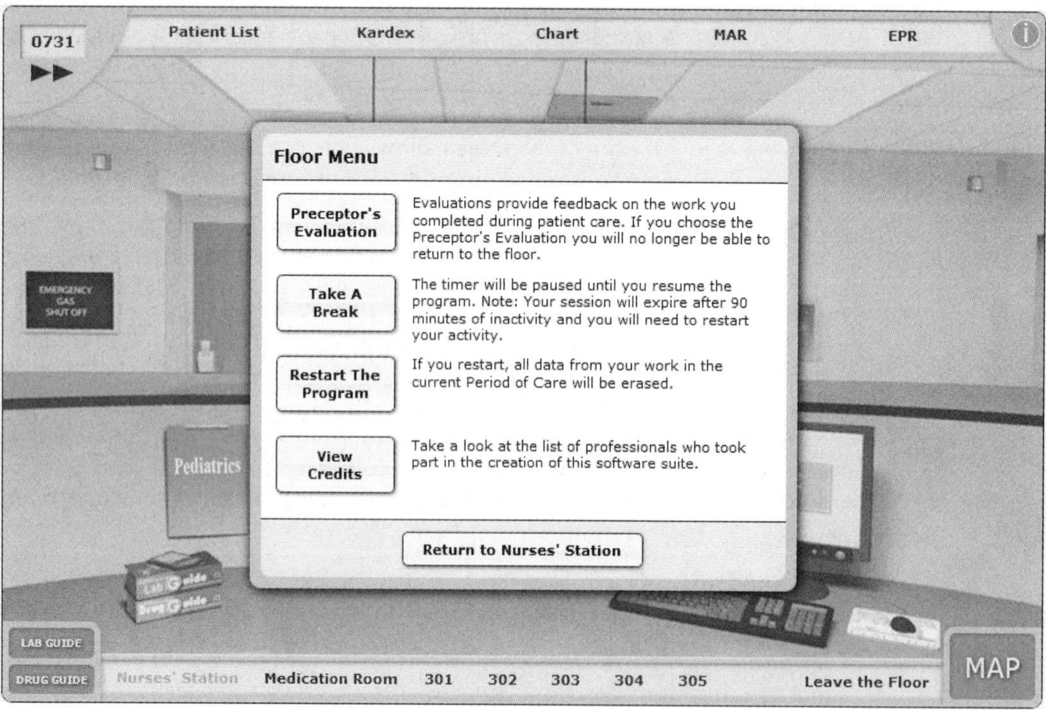

■ HOW TO PREPARE MEDICATIONS

From the Nurses' Station or the patient's room, you can access the Medication Room by clicking on the icon in the tool bar at the bottom of your screen to the left of the patient room numbers.

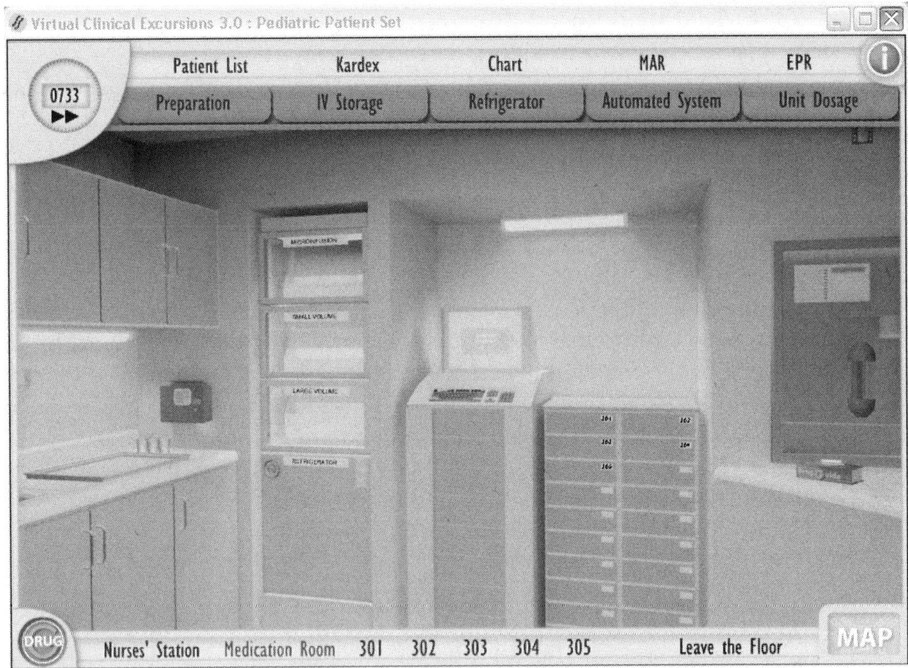

In the Medication Room you have access to the following (from left to right):

- A preparation area is located on the counter under the cabinets. To begin the medication preparation process, click on the tray on the counter or click on the **Preparation** icon at the top of the screen. The next screen leads you through a specific sequence (called the Preparation Wizard) to prepare medications one at a time for administration to a patient. However, no medication has been selected at this time. We will do this while working with a patient in **A Detailed Tour**. To exit this screen, click on **View Medication Room**.

- To the right of the cabinets (and above the refrigerator), IV storage bins are provided. Click on the bins themselves or on the **IV Storage** icon at the top of the screen. The bins are labeled **Microinfusion**, **Small Volume**, and **Large Volume**. Click on an individual bin to see a list of its contents. If you needed to prepare an IV medication at this time, you could click on the medication and its label would appear to the right under the patient's name. (*Note:* You can **Open** and **Close** any medication label by clicking the appropriate icon.) Next, you would click **Put Medication on Tray**. If you ever change your mind or decide that you have put the incorrect medication on the tray, you can reverse your actions by highlighting the medication on the tray and then clicking **Put Medication in Bin**. Click **Close Bin** in the right bottom corner to exit. **View Medication Room** brings you back to a full view of the entire room.

- A refrigerator is located under the IV storage bins to hold any medications that must be stored below room temperature. Click on the refrigerator door or on the **Refrigerator** icon at the top of the screen. Then click on the close-up view of the door to access the medications. When you are finished, click **Close Door** and then **View Medication Room**.

- To prepare controlled substances, click the **Automated System** icon at the top of the screen or click the computer monitor located to the right of the IV storage bins. A login screen will appear; your name and password are automatically filled in. Click **Login**. Select the patient for whom you wish to access medications; then select the correct medication drawer to open (they are stored alphabetically). Click **Open Drawer**, highlight the proper medication, and choose **Put Medication on Tray**. When you are finished, click **Close Drawer** and then **View Medication Room**.

- Next to the Automated System is a set of drawers identified by patient room number. To access these, click on the drawers or on the **Unit Dosage** icon at the top of the screen. This provides a close-up view of the drawers. To open a drawer, click on the room number of the patient you are working with. Next, click on the medication you would like to prepare for the patient, and a label will appear to the right, listing the medication strength, units, and dosage per unit. To exit, click **Close Drawer**; then click **View Medication Room**.

At any time, you can learn about a medication you wish to prepare for a patient by clicking on the **Drug** icon in the bottom left corner of the medication room screen or by clicking the **Drug Guide** book on the counter to the right of the unit dosage drawers. The **Drug Guide** provides information about the medications commonly included in nursing drug handbooks. Nutritional supplements and maintenance intravenous fluid preparations are not included. Highlight a medication in the alphabetical list; relevant information about the drug will appear in the screen below. To exit, click **Return to Medication Room**.

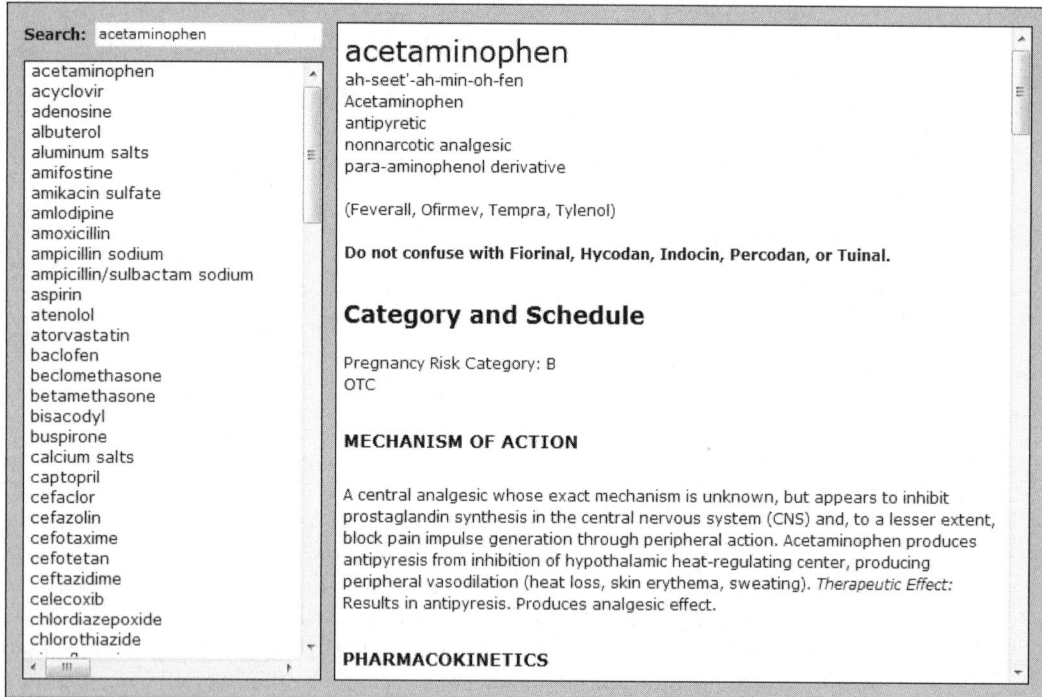

To access the MAR from the Medication Room and to review the medications ordered for a patient, click on the **MAR** icon located in the tool bar at the top of your screen and then click on the correct tab for your patient's room number. You may also click the **Review MAR** icon in the tool bar at the bottom of your screen from inside each medication storage area.

After you have chosen and prepared medications, go to the patient's room to administer them by clicking on the room number in the bottom tool bar. Inside the patient's room, click **Patient Care** and then **Medication Administration** and follow the proper administration sequence.

■ PRECEPTOR'S EVALUATIONS

When you have finished a session, click on **Leave the Floor** to go to the Floor Menu. At this point, you can click on the top icon (**Look at Your Preceptor's Evaluation**) to receive a scorecard that provides feedback on the work you completed during patient care.

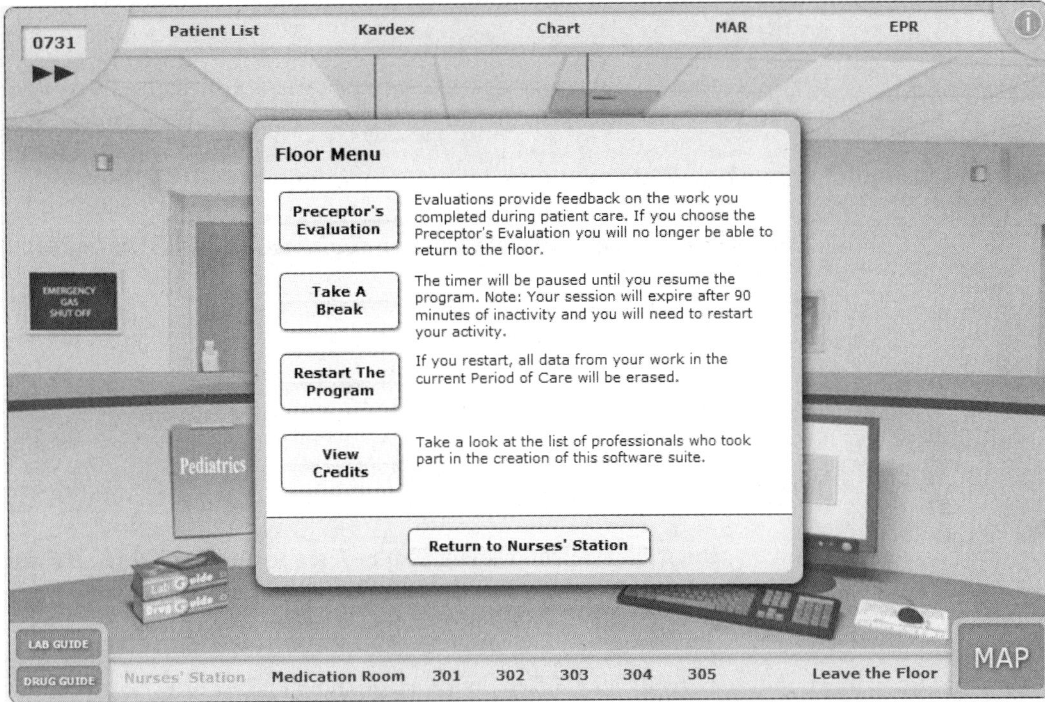

Evaluations are available for each patient you selected when you signed in for the current period of care. Click on the **Medication Scorecard** icon to see an example.

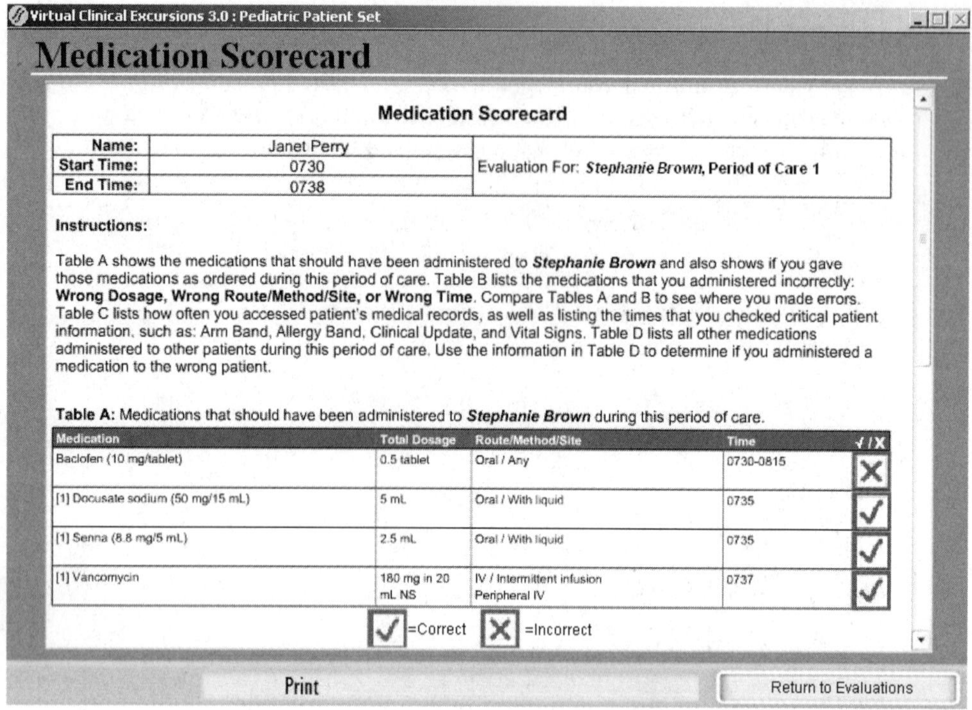

Medication	Total Dosage	Route/Method/Site	Time	✓/X
Baclofen (10 mg/tablet)	0.5 tablet	Oral / Any	0730-0815	X
[1] Docusate sodium (50 mg/15 mL)	5 mL	Oral / With liquid	0735	✓
[1] Senna (8.8 mg/5 mL)	2.5 mL	Oral / With liquid	0735	✓
[1] Vancomycin	180 mg in 20 mL NS	IV / Intermittent infusion Peripheral IV	0737	✓

The scorecard compares the medications you administered to a patient during a period of care with what should have been administered. Table A lists the correct medications. Table B lists any medications that were administered incorrectly.

Remember, not every medication listed on the MAR should necessarily be given. For example, a patient might have an allergy to a drug that was ordered, or a medication might have been improperly transcribed to the MAR. Predetermined medication "errors" embedded within the program challenge you to exercise critical thinking skills and professional judgment when deciding to administer a medication, just as you would in a real hospital. Use all your available resources, such as the patient's chart and the MAR, to make your decision.

Table C lists the resources that were available to assist you in medication administration. It also documents whether and when you accessed these resources. For example, did you check the patient armband or perform a check of vital signs? If so, when?

You can click **Print** to get a copy of this report if needed. When you have finished reviewing the scorecard, click **Return to Evaluations** and then **Return to Menu**.

■ FLOOR MAP

To get a general sense of your location within the hospital, you can click on the **Map** icon found in the lower right corner of most of the screens in the *Virtual Clinical Excursions—Pediatrics* program. (*Note:* If you are following this quick tour step by step, you will need to **Restart the Program** from the Floor Menu, sign in again, and go to the Nurses' Station to access the map.) When you click the **Map** icon, a floor map appears, showing the layout of the floor you are currently on, as well as a directory of the patients and services on that floor. As you move your cursor over the directory list, the location of each room is highlighted on the map (and vice versa). The floor map can be accessed from the Nurses' Station, Medication Room, and each patient's room.

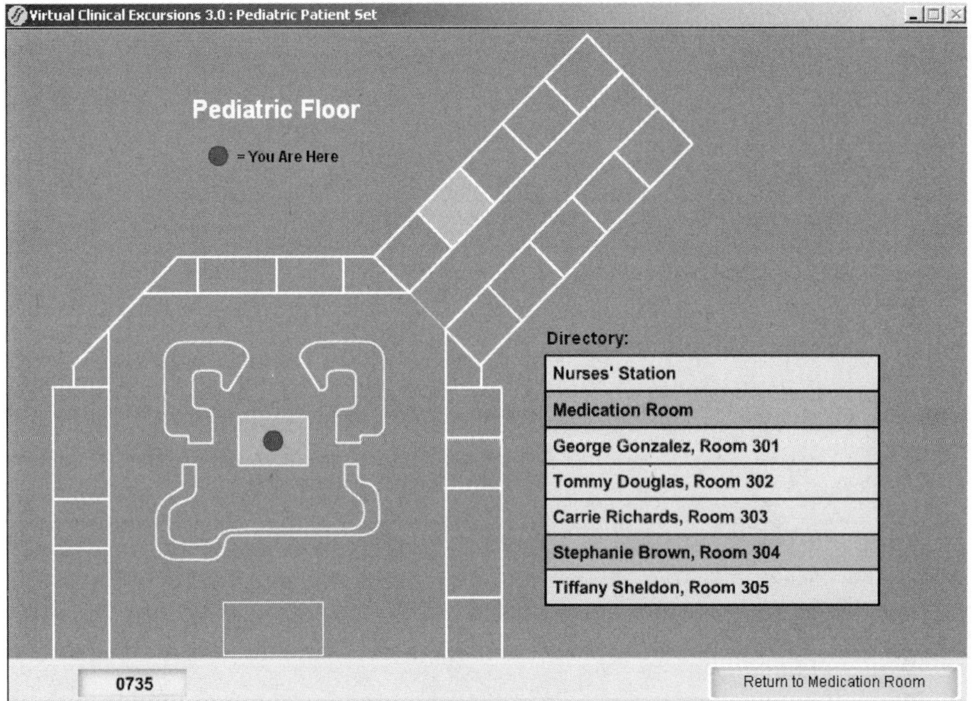

A DETAILED TOUR

If you wish to more thoroughly understand the capabilities of *Virtual Clinical Excursions— Pediatrics*, take a detailed tour by completing the following section. During this tour, we will work with a specific patient to introduce you to all the different components and learning opportunities available within the software.

■ WORKING WITH A PATIENT

Sign in for Period of Care 1 (0730-0815). From the Patient List, select Stephanie Brown in Room 304; however, do not go to the Nurses' Station yet.

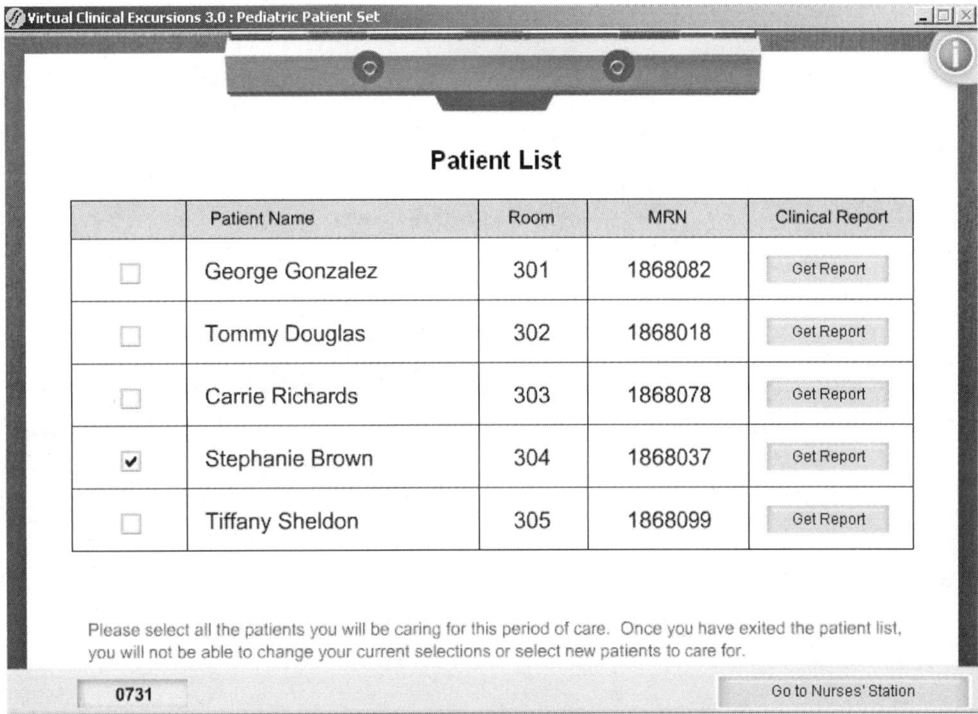

■ REPORT

In hospitals, when one shift ends and another begins, the outgoing nurse who attended a patient will give a verbal and sometimes a written summary of that patient's condition to the incoming nurse who will assume care for the patient. This summary is called a report and is an important source of data to provide an overview of a patient. Your first task is to get the clinical report on Stephanie Brown. To do this, click **Get Report** in the far right column in this patient's row. From a brief review of this summary, identify the problems and areas of concern that you will need to address for this patient.

When you have finished noting any areas of concern, click on **Go to Nurses' Station**.

■ CHARTS

You can access Stephanie Brown's chart from the Nurses' Station or from the patient's room (304). From the Nurses' Station, click on the chart rack or on the **Chart** icon in the tool bar at the top of your screen. Next, click on the chart labeled **304** to open the medical record for Stephanie Brown. Click on the **Emergency Department** tab to view a record of why this patient was admitted.

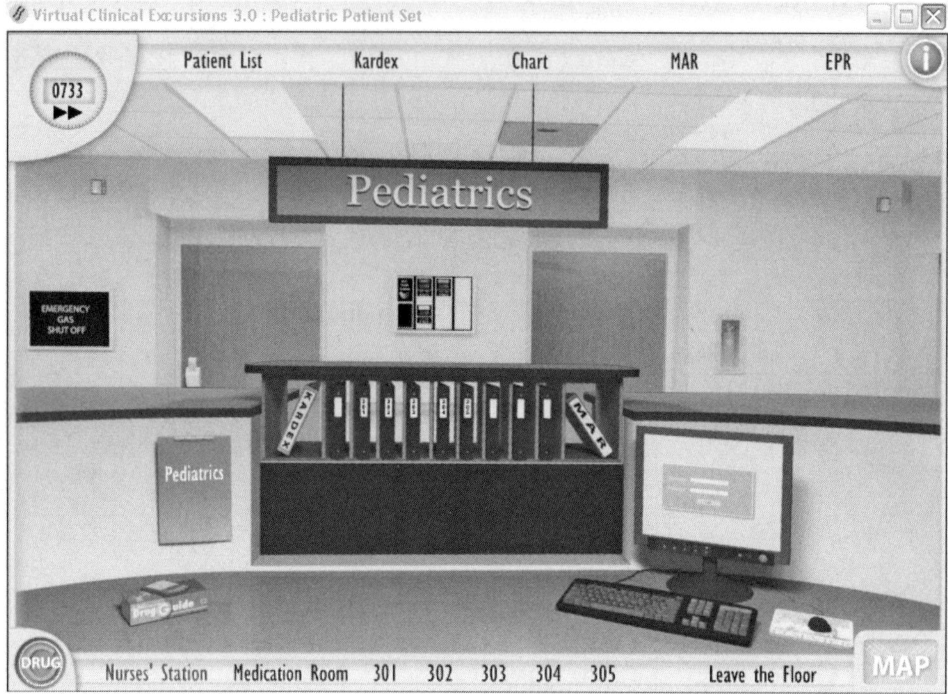

How many days has Stephanie Brown been in the hospital?

What tests were done upon her arrival in the Emergency Department and why?

What was her reason for admission?

You should also click on **Diagnostic Reports** to learn what additional tests or procedures were performed and when. Finally, review the **Nursing Admission** and **History and Physical** to learn about the health history of this patient. When you are done reviewing the chart, click **Return to Nurses' Station**.

■ MEDICATIONS

Open the Medication Administration Record (MAR) by clicking on the **MAR** icon in the tool bar at the top of your screen. *Remember:* The MAR automatically opens to the first occupied room number on the floor—which is not necessarily your patient's room number! Since you need to access Stephanie Brown's MAR, click on tab **304** (her room number). Always make sure you are giving the *Right Drug to the Right Patient!*

Examine the list of medications ordered for Stephanie Brown. In the table below, list the medications that need to be given during this period of care (0730-0815). For each medication, note the dosage, route, and time to be given.

Time	Medication	Dosage	Route

Click on **Return to Nurses' Station**. Next, click on **304** on the bottom tool bar and then verify that you are indeed in Stephanie Brown's room. Select **Clinical Alerts** (the icon to the right of Initial Observations) to check for any emerging data that might affect your medication administration priorities. Next, go to the patient's chart (click on the **Chart** icon; then click on **304**). When the chart opens, select the **Physician's Orders** tab.

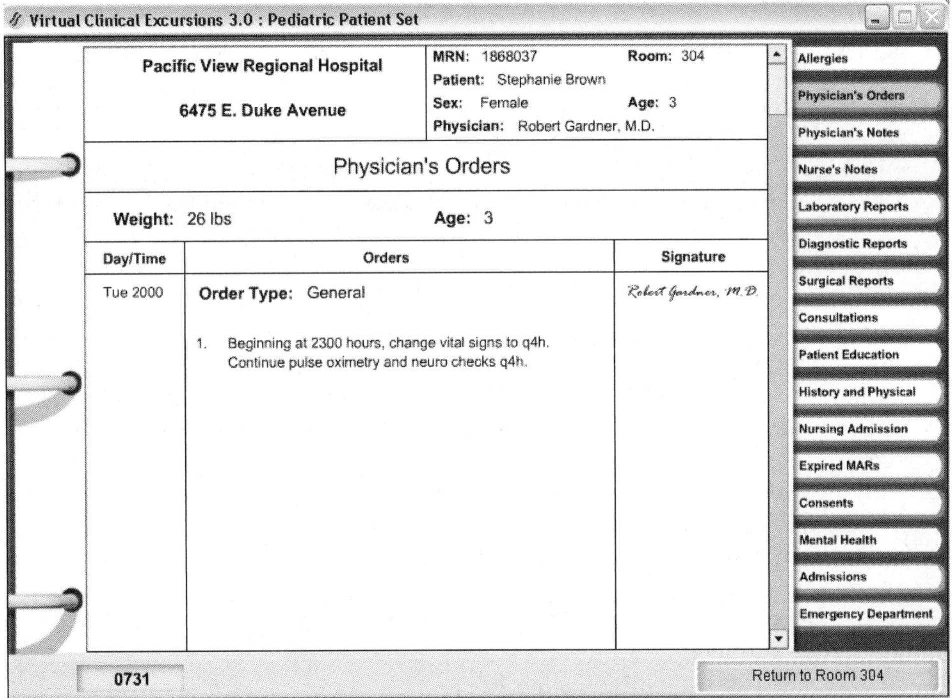

Review the orders. Have any new medications been ordered? Return to the MAR (click **Return to Room 304**; then click **MAR**). Verify that any new medications have been correctly transcribed to the MAR. Mistakes are sometimes made in the transcription process in the hospital setting, and it is sound practice to double-check any new order.

Are there any patient assessments you will need to perform before administering these medications? If so, return to Room 304 and click on **Patient Care** and then **Physical Assessment** to complete those assessments before proceeding.

Now click on the **Medication Room** icon in the tool bar at the bottom of your screen to locate and prepare the medications for Stephanie Brown.

In the Medication Room, you must access the medications for Stephanie Brown from the specific dispensing system in which each medication is stored. Locate each medication that needs to be given in this time period and click on **Put Medication on Tray** as appropriate. (*Hint:* Look in **Unit Dosage** drawer first.) When you are finished, click on **Close Drawer** and then on **View Medication Room**. Now click on the medication tray on the counter on the left side of the medication room screen to begin preparing the medications you have selected. (*Remember:* You can also click **Preparation** in the tool bar at top of the screen.)

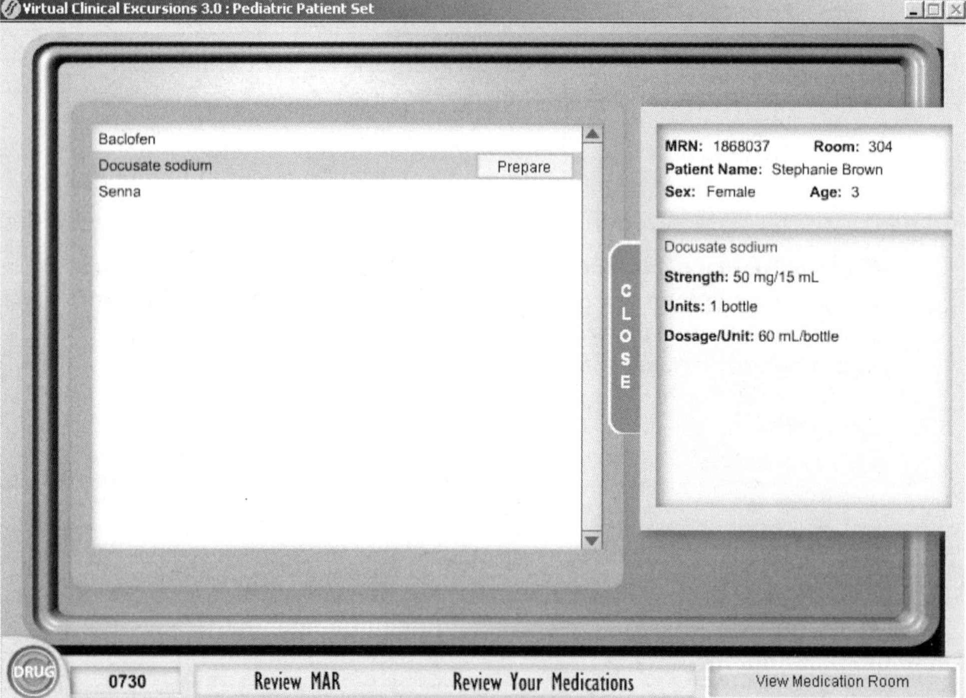

In the preparation area, you should see a list of the medications you put on the tray in the previous steps. Click on the first medication and then click **Prepare**. Follow the onscreen instructions of the Preparation Wizard, providing any data requested. As an example, let's follow the preparation process for docusate sodium, one of the medications due to be administered to Stephanie Brown during this period of care. To begin, click to select **Docusate sodium**; then click **Prepare**. Now work through the Preparation Wizard sequence as detailed below:

> Amount of medication in the bottle: 60 mL.
> Enter the amount of medication you will draw up into a syringe: **5** mL.
> Click **Next**.
> Select the patient you wish to set aside the medication for: **Room 304, Stephanie Brown**.
> Click **Finish**.
> Click **Return to Medication Room**.

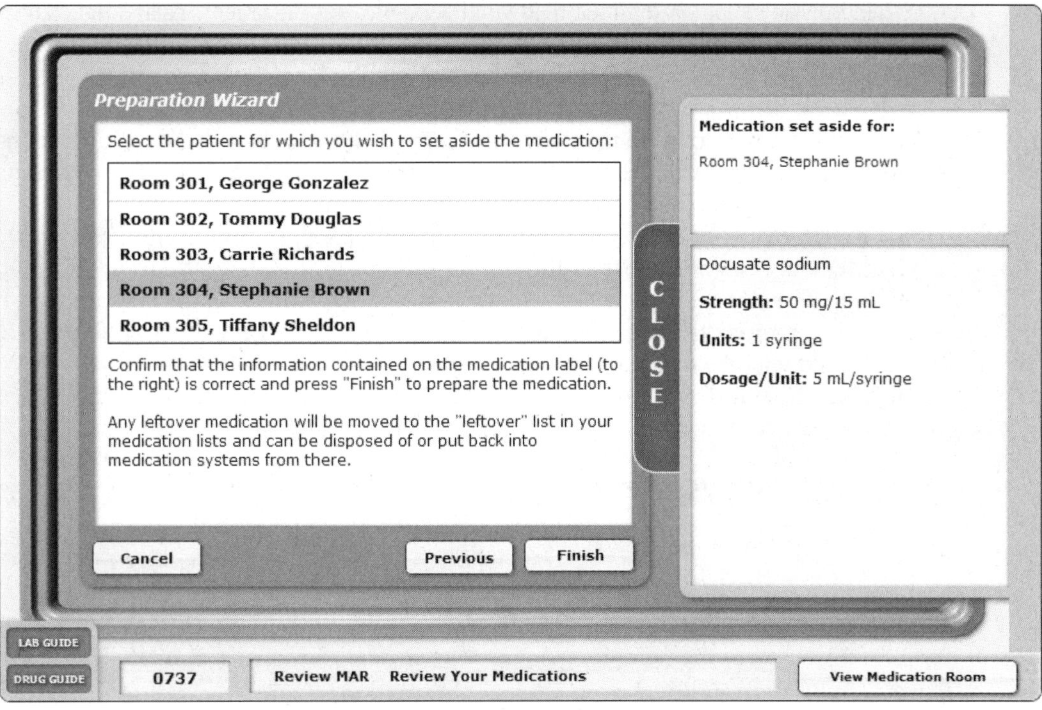

Follow this same basic process for the other medications due to be administered to Stephanie Brown during this period of care. (*Hint:* Look in **IV Storage** and **Automated System**.)

PREPARATION WIZARD EXCEPTIONS

- Some medications in *Virtual Clinical Excursions—Pediatrics* are preprepared by the pharmacy (e.g., IV antibiotics) and taken to the patient room as a whole. This is common practice in most hospitals.
- Blood products are not administered by students through the *Virtual Clinical Excursions—Pediatrics* simulations since blood administration follows specific protocols not covered in this program.
- The *Virtual Clinical Excursions—Pediatrics* simulations do not allow for mixing more than one type of medication, such as regular and Lente insulins, in the same syringe. In the clinical setting, when multiple types of insulin are ordered for a patient, the regular insulin is drawn up first, followed by the longer-acting insulin. Insulin is always administered in a special unit-marked syringe.

Now return to Room 304 (click on **304** on the bottom tool bar) to administer Stephanie Brown's medications.

At any time during the medication administration process, you can perform a further review of systems, take vital signs, check information contained within the chart, or verify patient identity and allergies. Inside Stephanie Brown's room, click **Take Vital Signs**. (*Note:* These findings change over time to reflect the temporal changes you would find in a patient similar to Stephanie Brown.)

When you have gathered all the data you need, click on **Patient Care** and then select **Medication Administration**. Any medications you prepared in the previous steps should be listed on the left side of your screen. Let's continue the administration process with the vancomycin ordered for Stephanie Brown. Click to highlight **Vancomycin** in the list of medications. Next, click on the down arrow to the right of **Select** and choose **Administer** from the drop-down menu. This will activate the Administration Wizard. Complete the Wizard sequence as follows:

- Route: **IV**
- Method: **Intermittent Infusion**
- Site: **Peripheral IV**
- Click **Administer to Patient** arrow.
- Would you like to document this administration in the MAR? **Yes**
- Click **Finish** arrow.

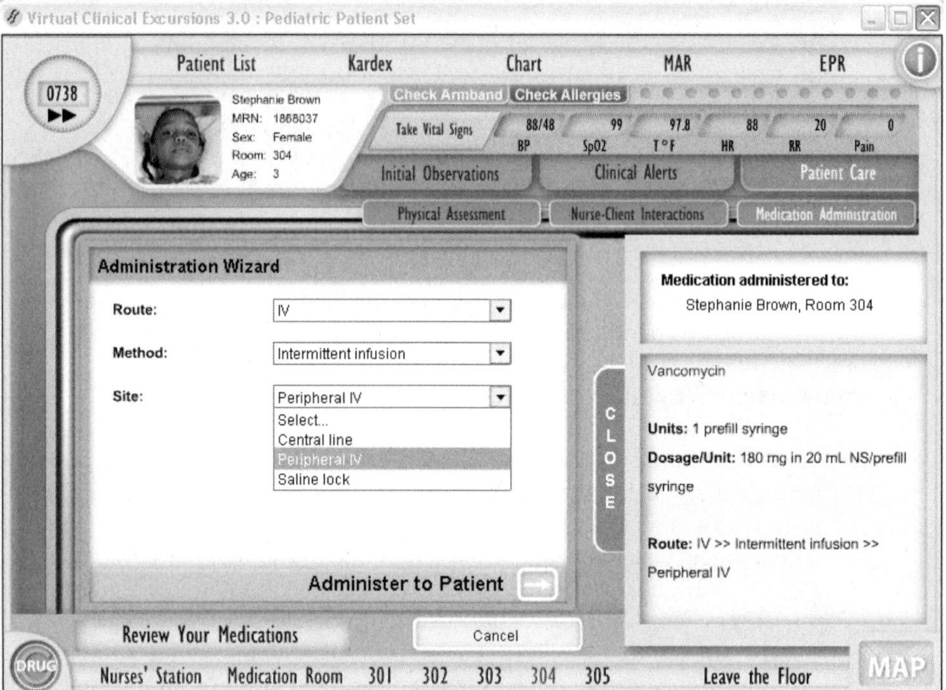

Your selections are recorded by a tracking system and evaluated on a Medication Scorecard stored under Preceptor's Evaluations. This scorecard can be viewed, printed, and given to your instructor. To access the Preceptor's Evaluations, click on **Leave the Floor**. When the Floor Menu appears, select **Look at Your Preceptor's Evaluation**. Then click on **Medication Scorecard** inside the box with Stephanie Brown's name (see example on the following page).

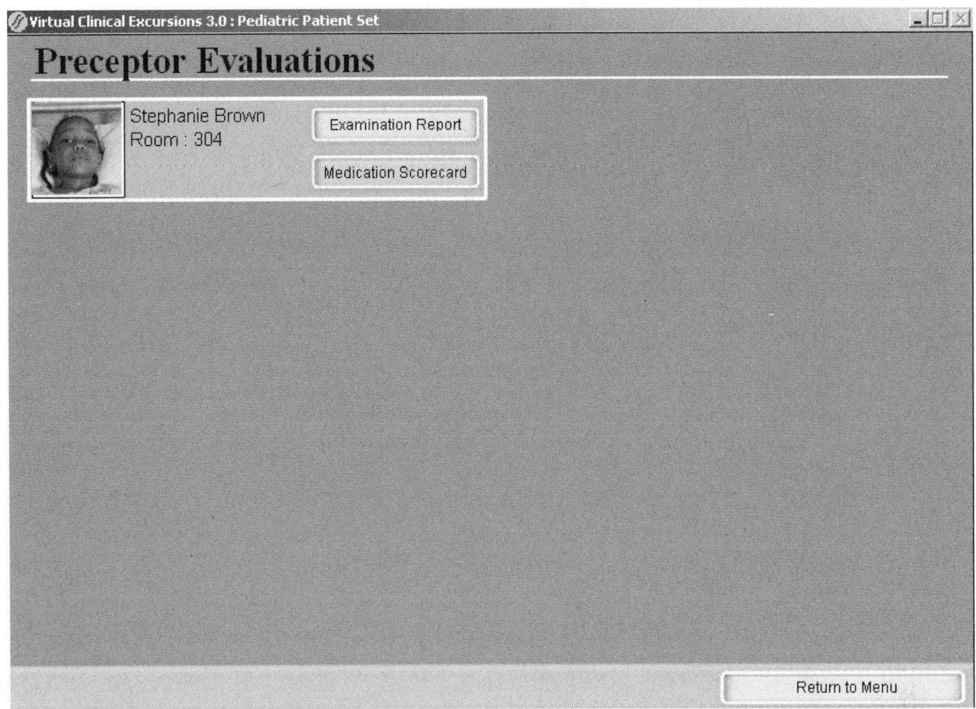

■ MEDICATION SCORECARD

- First, review Table A. Was vancomycin given correctly? Did you give the other medications as ordered?
- Table B shows you which (if any) medications you gave incorrectly.
- Table C addresses the resources used for Stephanie Brown. Did you access the patient's chart, MAR, EPR, or Kardex as needed to make safe medication administration decisions?
- Did you check the patient's armband to verify her identity? Did you check whether your patient had any known allergies to medications? Were vital signs taken?

When you have finished reviewing the scorecard, click **Return to Evaluations** and then **Return to Menu**.

■ VITAL SIGNS

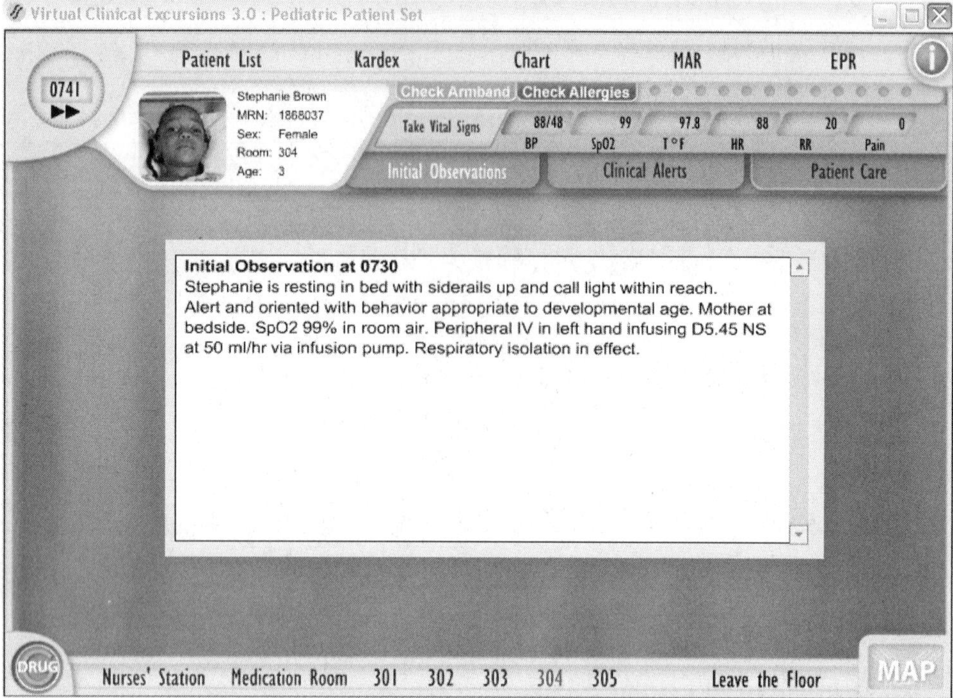

Vital signs, often considered the traditional "signs of life," include body temperature, heart rate, respiratory rate, blood pressure, oxygen saturation of the blood, and pain level.

Inside Stephanie Brown's room, click **Take Vital Signs**. (*Note:* If you are following this detailed tour step by step, you will need to **Restart the Program** from the Floor Menu, sign in again for Period of Care 1, and navigate to Room 304.) Collect vital signs for this patient and record them below. Note the time at which you collected each of these data. (*Remember:* You can take vital signs at any time. The data change over time to reflect the temporal changes you would find in a patient similar to Stephanie Brown.)

Vital Signs	Findings/Time
Blood pressure	
O$_2$ saturation	
Temperature	
Heart rate	
Respiratory rate	
Pain rating	

After you are done, click on the **EPR** icon located in the tool bar at the top of the screen. Your username and password are automatically provided. Click on **Login** to enter the EPR. To access Stephanie's records, click on the down arrow next to Patient and choose her room number, **304**. Select **Vital Signs** as the category. Next, in the empty time column on the far right, record the vital signs data you just collected in Stephanie's room. If you need help with this process, refer to the *Electronic Patient Record (EPR)* section of **A Quick Tour**. Now compare these findings with the data you collected earlier for this patient's vital signs. Use these earlier findings to establish a baseline for each of the vital signs.

    a.   Are any of the data you collected significantly different from the baseline for a particular vital sign?

       Circle One: Yes   No

    b.   If "Yes," which data are different?

■ PHYSICAL ASSESSMENT

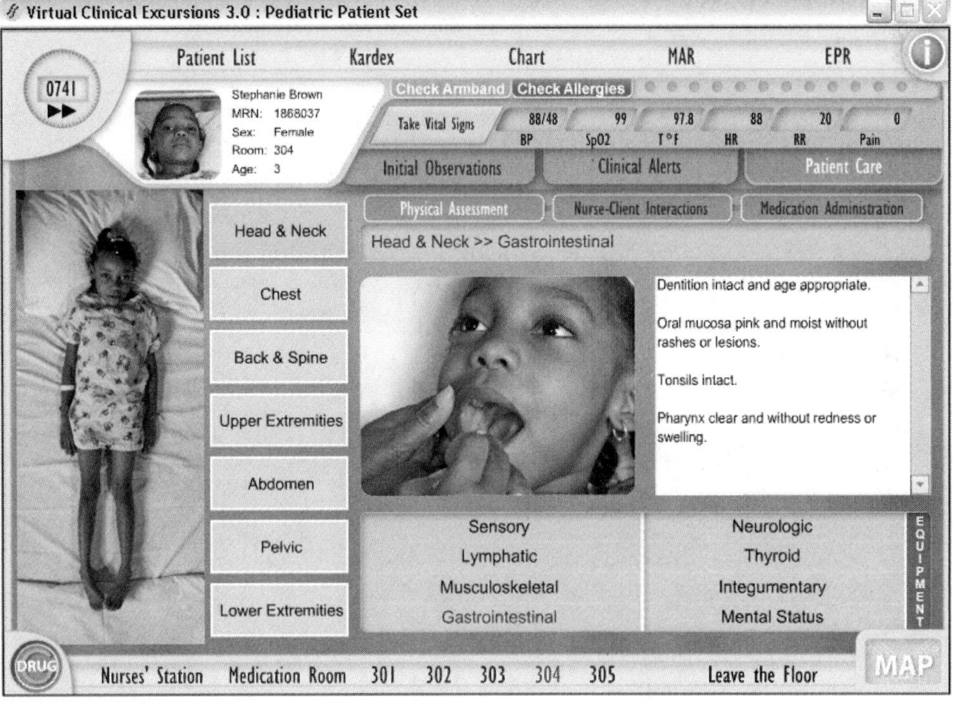

After you have finished examining the EPR for vital signs, click **Exit EPR** to return to Room 304. Click **Patient Care** and then **Physical Assessment**. Think about the information you received in the report at the beginning of this shift, as well as what you may have learned about this patient from the chart. Based on this, what area(s) of examination should you pay most attention to at this time? Is there any equipment you should be monitoring? Conduct a physical assessment of the body areas and systems that you consider priorities for Stephanie Brown. For example, select **Head & Neck**; then click on and assess **Sensory** and **Lymphatic**. Complete any other assessment(s) you think are necessary at this time. In the following table, record the data you collected during this examination.

Area of Examination	Findings
Head & Neck Sensory	
Head & Neck Lymphatic	

After you have finished collecting these data, return to the EPR. Compare the data that were already in the record with those you just collected.

a. Are any of the data you collected significantly different from the baselines for this patient?

Circle One: Yes   No

b. If "Yes," which data are different?

■ NURSE-CLIENT INTERACTIONS

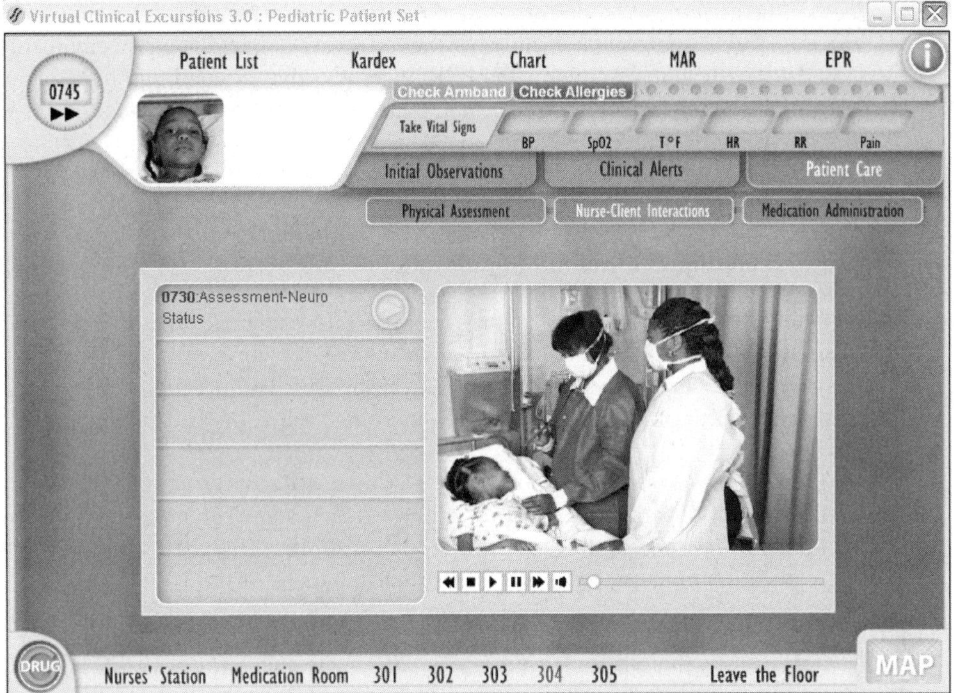

Click on **Patient Care** from inside Stephanie Brown's room (304). Now click on **Nurse-Client Interactions** to access a short video titled **Assessment—Neuro Status**, which is available for viewing at or after 0730 (based on the virtual clock in the upper left corner of your screen; see *Note* below). To begin the video, click on the white arrow next to its title. You will observe a nurse explaining her actions to Stephanie's mother. There are many variations of nursing practice, some exemplifying "best" practice and some not. Note whether the nurse in this interaction displays professional behavior and compassionate care. Are her words congruent with what is going on with the patient? Does this interaction "feel right" to you? If not, how would you handle this situation differently? Explain.

Note: If the video you wish to view is not listed, this means you have not yet reached the correct virtual time to view that video. Check the virtual clock; you may return to access the video once its designated time has occurred—as long as you do so within the same period of care. Or you can click on the fast-forward icon within the virtual clock to advance the time by 2-minute intervals. You will then need to click again on **Patient Care** and **Nurse-Client Interactions** to refresh the screen.

At least one Nurse-Client Interactions video is available during each period of care. Viewing these videos can help you learn more about what is occurring with a patient at a certain time and also prompt you to discern between nurse communications that are ideal and those that need improvement. Compassionate care and the ability to communicate clearly are essential components of delivering quality nursing care, and it is during your clinical time that you will begin to refine these skills.

■ COLLECTING AND EVALUATING DATA

Each of the activities you perform in the Patient Care environment generates a significant amount of assessment data. Remember that after you collect data, you can record your findings in the EPR. You can also review the EPR, patient's chart, videos, and MAR at any time. You will get plenty of practice collecting and then evaluating data in context of the patient's course.

Now, here's an important question for you:

> Did the previous sequence of exercises provide the most efficient way to assess Stephanie Brown?

For example, you went to the patient's room to get vital signs, then back to the EPR to enter data and compare your findings with extant data. Next, you went back to the patient's room to do a physical examination, then again back to the EPR to enter and review data. If this back-and-forth process of data collection and recording seemed inefficient, remember the following:

- Plan all of your nursing activities to maximize efficiency, while at the same time optimizing the quality of patient care. (Think about what data you might need before performing certain tasks. For example, do you need to check a heart rate before administering a cardiac medication or check an IV site before starting an infusion?)

- You collect a tremendous amount of data when you work with a patient. Very few people can accurately remember all these data for more than a few minutes. Develop efficient assessment skills, and record data as soon as possible after collecting them.

- Assessment data are only the starting point for the nursing process.

Make a clear distinction between these first exercises and how you actually provide nursing care. These initial exercises were designed to involve you actively in the use of different software components. This workbook focuses on sensible practices for implementing the nursing process in ways that ensure the highest-quality care of patients.

Most important, remember that a human being changes through time, and that these changes include both the physical and psychosocial facets of a person as a living organism. Think about this for a moment. Some patients may change physically in a very short time (a patient with emerging myocardial infarction) or more slowly (a patient with a chronic illness). Patients' overall physical and psychosocial conditions may improve or deteriorate. They may have effective coping skills and familial support, or they may feel alone and full of despair. In fact, each individual is a complex mix of physical and psychosocial elements, and at least some of these elements usually change through time.

Thus it is crucial that you *DO NOT* think of the nursing process as a simple one-time, five-step procedure consisting of assessment, nursing diagnosis, planning, implementation, and evaluation. Rather, the nursing process should be utilized as a creative and systematic approach to delivering nursing care. Furthermore, because all living organisms are constantly changing, we must apply the nursing process over and over. Each time we follow the nursing process for an individual patient, we refine our understanding of that patient's physical and psychosocial conditions based on collection and analysis of many different types of data. *Virtual Clinical Excursions—Pediatrics* will help you develop both the creativity and the systematic approach needed to become a nurse who is equipped to deliver the highest-quality care to all patients.

REDUCING MEDICATION ERRORS

Earlier in the detailed tour, you learned the basic steps of medication preparation and administration. The following simulations will allow you to practice those skills further—with an increased emphasis on reducing medication errors by using the Medication Scorecard to evaluate your work.

Sign in to work at Pacific View Regional Hospital for Period of Care 2. (*Note:* If you are already working with another patient or during another period of care, click on **Leave the Floor** and then **Restart the Program**; then sign in.)

From the Patient List, select Stephanie Brown. Then click on **Go to Nurses' Station**. Complete the following steps to prepare and administer medications to Stephanie Brown.

- Click on **Medication Room** on the tool bar at the bottom of your screen.
- Click on **MAR** and then on tab **304** to determine prn medications that have been ordered for Stephanie Brown. (*Note:* You may click on **Review MAR** at any time to verify the correct medication order. Always remember to check the patient name on the MAR to make sure you have the correct patient's record. You must click on the correct room number tab within the MAR.) Click on **Return to Medication Room** after reviewing the correct MAR.
- Click on **Unit Dosage** (or on the Unit Dosage cabinet); from the close-up view, click on drawer **304**.
- Select the medications you would like to administer. After each selection, click **Put Medication on Tray**. When you are finished selecting medications, click **Close Drawer** and then **View Medication Room**.
- Click on **Automated System** (or on the Automated System unit itself). Click **Login**.
- On the next screen, specify the correct patient and drawer location.
- Select the medication you would like to administer and click on **Put Medication on Tray**. Repeat this process if you wish to administer other medications from the Automated System.
- When you are finished, click **Close Drawer** and **View Medication Room**.
- From the Medication Room, click on **Preparation** (or on the preparation tray).
- From the list of medications on your tray, highlight the correct medication to administer and click **Prepare**.
- This activates the Preparation Wizard. Supply any requested information; then click **Next**.
- Now select the correct patient to receive this medication and click **Finish**.
- Repeat the previous three steps until all medications that you want to administer are prepared.
- You can click on **Review Your Medications** and then on **Return to Medication Room** when ready. Once you are back in the Medication Room, go directly to Stephanie Brown's room by clicking on **304** at bottom of screen.
- Inside the patient's room, administer the medication, utilizing the six rights of medication administration. After you have collected the appropriate assessment data and are ready for administration, click **Patient Care** and then **Medication Administration**. Verify that the correct patient and medication(s) appear in the left-hand window. Highlight the first medication you wish to administer; then click the down arrow next to Select. From the drop-down menu, select **Administer** and complete the Administration Wizard by providing any information requested. When the Wizard stops asking for information, click **Administer to Patient**. Specify **Yes** when asked whether this administration should be recorded in the MAR. Finally, click **Finish**.

■ SELF-EVALUATION

Now let's see how you did during your medication administration!

- Click on **Leave the Floor** at the bottom of your screen. From the Floor Menu, select **Look at Your Preceptor's Evaluation**. Then click on **Medication Scorecard**.

The following exercises will help you identify medication errors, investigate possible reasons for these errors, and reduce or prevent medication errors in the future.

1. Start by examining Table A. These are the medications you should have given to Stephanie Brown during this period of care. If each of the medications in Table A has a ✓ by it, then you made no errors. Congratulations!

If any medication has an X by it, then you made one or more medication errors.

Compare Tables A and B to determine which of the following types of errors you made: Wrong Dose, Wrong Route/Method/Site, or Wrong Time. Follow these steps:
   a. Find medications in Table A that were given incorrectly.
   b. Now see if those same medications are in Table B, which shows what you actually administered to Stephanie Brown.
   c. Comparing Tables A and B, match the Strength, Dose, Route/Method/Site, and Time for each medication you administered incorrectly.
   d. Then, using the form below, list the medications given incorrectly and mark the errors you made for each medication.

Medication	Strength	Dosage	Route	Method	Site	Time
	❑	❑	❑	❑	❑	❑
	❑	❑	❑	❑	❑	❑
	❑	❑	❑	❑	❑	❑
	❑	❑	❑	❑	❑	❑

2. To help you reduce future medication errors, consider the following list of possible reasons for errors.

- Did not check drug against MAR for correct medication, correct dose, correct patient, correct route, correct time, correct documentation.
- Did not check drug dose against MAR three times.
- Did not open the unit dose package in the patient's room.
- Did not correctly identify the patient using two identifiers.
- Did not administer the drug on time.
- Did not verify patient allergies.
- Did not check the patient's current condition or vital sign parameters.
- Did not consider why the patient would be receiving this drug.
- Did not question why the drug was in the patient's drawer.
- Did not check the physician's order and/or check with the pharmacist when there was a question about the drug or dose.
- Did not verify that no adverse effects had occurred from a previous dose.

Based on the list of possibilities you just reviewed, determine how you made each error and record the reason in the form below:

Medication	Reason for Error

3. Look again at Table B. Are there medications listed that are not in Table A? If so, you gave a medication to Stephanie Brown that she should not have received. Complete the following exercises to help you understand how such an error might have been made.

   a. Perhaps you gave a medication that was on Stephanie Brown's MAR for this period of care, without recognizing that a change had occurred in the patient's condition, which should have caused you to reconsider. Review patient records as necessary and complete the following form:

Medication	Possible Reasons Not to Give This Medication

   b. Another possibility is that you gave Stephanie Brown a medication that should have been given at a different time. Check her MAR and complete the form below to determine whether you made a Wrong Time error:

Medication	Given to Stephanie Brown at What Time	Should Have Been Given at What Time

c. Maybe you gave another patient's medication to Stephanie Brown. In this case, you made a Wrong Patient error. Check the MARs of other patients and use the form below to determine whether you made this type of error:

Medication	Given to Stephanie Brown	Should Have Been Given to

4. The Medication Scorecard provides some other interesting sources of information. For example, if there is a medication selected for Stephanie Brown but it was not given to her, there will be an X by that medication in Table A, but it will not appear in Table B. In that case, you might have given this medication to some other patient, which is another type of Wrong Patient error. To investigate further, look at Table D, which lists the medications you gave to other patients. See whether you can find any medications ordered for Stephanie Brown that were given to another patient by mistake. However, before you make any decisions, be sure to cross-check the MAR for other patients because the same medication may have been ordered for multiple patients. Use the following form to record your findings:

Medication	Should Have Been Given to Stephanie Brown	Given by Mistake to

5. Now take some time to review the medication exercises you just completed. Use the form below to create an overall analysis of what you have learned. Once again, record each of the medication errors you made, including the type of each error. Then, for each error you made, indicate specifically what you would do differently to prevent this type of error from occurring again.

Medication	Type of Error	Error Prevention Tactic

Submit this form to your instructor if required as a graded assignment, or simply use these exercises to improve your understanding of medication errors and how to reduce them.

Name: ____   Date: _______________________

LESSON 1

Understanding Head Injury

Reading Assignments:
Hockenberry: Wong's Essentials of Pediatric Nursing, 10th edition (Chapters 19 and 27)
Hockenberry: Wong's Nursing Care of Infants and Children, 10th edition (Chapter 32)

Patient: Tommy Douglas, Room 302

Objectives:

1. Evaluate the pathophysiology related to acute head trauma in children.
2. Participate in the care of a comatose child.
3. Review medications given to a child who has experienced a head injury.

Exercise 1

Writing Activity

20 minutes

1. What are the clinical symptoms of increased intracranial pressure (ICP) in a child Tommy Douglas' age and in his condition?

2. List three causes of ICP.

3. What components make up the cranium's total volume?

4. Which of the following vital sign changes are associated with brainstem injury following acute head trauma? Select all that apply.

   _______ Wide fluctuations in pulse

   _______ Widening pulse pressure

   _______ Extreme fluctuations in blood pressure

   _______ Elevated temperature

5. One of Tommy Douglas' patient problems is Potential for injury related to physical immobility, depressed sensorium, and intracranial pathology. List four nursing interventions for this patient problem specific to maintaining a stable ICP.

6. What is the expected outcome related to the patient problem presented in question 5?

Exercise 2

Virtual Hospital Activity

25 minutes

- Sign in to work at Pacific View Regional Hospital for Period of Care 1. (*Note:* If you are already in the virtual hospital from a previous exercise, click on **Leave the Floor** and then on **Restart the Program** to get to the sign-in window.)
- From the Patient List, select Tommy Douglas (Room 302).
- Click on **Go to Nurses' Station**.
- Click on **Chart** and then on **302**.
- Select the **Emergency Department** tab and review the Admission Notes.
- While in the chart, also click on and review the **Nurse's Notes** and the **History and Physical.**

1. What caused Tommy Douglas' head injury?

- Now click on **Expired MARs** and review Tommy Douglas' expired MAR for Sunday at 2300.
- Next, click on **Physician's Orders** and review orders written in the Emergency Department.
- For additional help with the following questions, consult the Drug Guide by first clicking on **Return to Nurses' Station** and then clicking either on the **Drug** icon in the lower left corner of the screen or on the Drug Guide itself on the counter.

2. Based on your knowledge of head injury, why did Tommy Douglas receive mannitol?

3. Describe the sequence of events from Tommy Douglas' admission to the Emergency Department to his admission to your unit. (*Hint:* For help, check the Nurse's Notes, Physician's Notes, and Physician's Orders sections of the chart.)

4. List three interventions specific to the treatment of a child with a head injury that were performed before Tommy Douglas' arrival on your unit.

Assessing the Patient with a Head Injury

Reading Assignments:
   Hockenberry: Wong's Essentials of Pediatric Nursing, 10th edition (Chapters 4 and 27)
   Hockenberry: Wong's Nursing Care of Infants and Children, 10th edition (Chapters 4 and 32)

Patient: Tommy Douglas, Room 302

Objectives:

1. Perform a neurologic assessment on a child who has experienced a head injury.
2. Participate in the care of a comatose child.

Exercise 1

Virtual Hospital Activity

35 minutes

- Sign in to work at Pacific View Regional Hospital for Period of Care 1. (*Note:* If you are already in the virtual hospital from a previous exercise, click on **Leave the Floor** and then on **Restart the Program** to get to the sign-in window.)
- From the Patient List, select Tommy Douglas (Room 302).
- Click on **Go to Nurses' Station**.
- Click on **Chart** and then on **302**.
- Click on **Emergency Department** and review the Admission Notes.
- Click on and review the **Nurse's Notes** and the **Physician's Notes**.

1. What are the major components of the Glasgow Coma Scale?

2. In the following table, briefly describe how each of these diagnostic tests is performed. Then provide a rationale for each test to explain its use in assessing the extent of Tommy Douglas' head injury. (*Hint:* See the diagnostic tests found in Tommy's medical record.)

Diagnostic Test	How Test Is Performed	Rationale for Test
Brain CT without contrast		
Skull radiograph		
Cervical spine radiograph		
Single-photon emission computed tomography (SPECT)		

Now let's assess Tommy Douglas' neurologic status over time since his admission to the Emergency Department. To do this, find neurologic assessment data in the virtual hospital resources listed below; then record your findings in the table as instructed in questions 3 and 4.

- In the patient's chart, click on **Emergency Department** and review the report for Sunday admission.
- Next, click on **Physician's Notes** and review the notes for Monday 0930 and Tuesday 1730.
- Click on **Return to Nurses' Station**.
- Select **EPR** and click on **Login**.
- Select **302** from the Patient drop-down menu and **Neurologic** from the Category drop-down menu.
- Review the neurologic findings for 0715 Wednesday.

3. In the table below, record the findings from your chart review of Tommy Douglas' neurologic status on Sunday, Monday, Tuesday, and Wednesday.

Neurologic Exam	Sunday Admission	Monday 0930	Tuesday 1730	Wednesday 0715
GCS: Total Score				
Pupils Right: Size				
Pupils Right: Reaction				
Pupils Left: Size				
Pupils Left: Reaction				
Cranial Nerves I-XII				
Orientation				
Perception and Cognition				
Mental Status				
Sensory				

- Click on **Exit EPR** and then on **Leave the Floor**.
- At the Floor Menu, select **Restart the Program**.
- Sign in for Period of Care 2.
- Again, select Tommy Douglas as your patient and click on **Go to Nurses' Station**.
- Now click on **EPR** and then on **Login**.
- Choose **302** from the Patient drop-down menu and **Neurologic** from the Category drop-down menu.
- Review the results of the neurologic assessment recorded on Wednesday at 0800.

4.

NEUROLOGIC ASSESSMENT

GLASGOW COMA SCALE				
Pupils	Right	Size		
		Reaction		
	Left	Size		
		Reaction		
Eyes open	Spontaneously	4		
	To speech	3		
	To pain	2		
	None	1		
Best motor response	Obeys commands	6		
	Localizes pain	5		
	Flexion withdrawal	4		
	Flexion abnormal	3		
	Extension	2		
	None	1		

++ = Brisk
+ = Sluggish
− = No reaction
C = Eye closed by swelling

Usually record best arm or age-appropriate response

Pupil scale (mm): 1, 2, 3, 4, 5, 6, 7, 8

Best response to auditory and/or visual stimulus	>2 years		<2 years
	Orientation	5	5 Smiles, listens, follows
	Confused	4	4 Cries, consolable
	Inappropriate words	3	3 Inappropriate persistent cry
	Incomprehensible words	2	2 Agitated, restless
	None	1	1 No response
	Endotracheal tube or trach	T	

COMA SCALE TOTAL

HAND GRIP:
Equal
Unequal
R_____L
Weakness

LOC:
Alert/oriented x4
Sleepy
Irritable
Comatose
Disoriented
Combative
Lethargic
Awake
Sleeping
Drowsy
Agitated

MUSCLE TONE:
Normal
Arching
Spastic
Flaccid
Weak
Decorticate
Decerebrate
Other _________

EYE MOVEMENT:
Normal
Nystagmus
Strabismus
Other _________

FONTANEL/WINDOW:
Soft
Flat
Sunken
Tense
Bulging
Closed
Other _________

MOOD/AFFECT:
Happy
Content
Quiet
Withdrawn
Sad
Flat
Hostile

Complete the Glasgow Coma Scale readings below, using the findings from Tommy Douglas' neurologic examination at 0800 Wednesday morning.

Pupils right: size: _______

Pupils right: reaction: _______

Pupils left: size: _______

Pupils left: reaction: _______

Eyes open: _______

Best motor response: _______

Best response to auditory and/or visual stimulus: _______

Endotracheal tube or trach:

____

Coma Scale total: _______

Hand grip: ___________

LOC: ___________

Muscle tone: ___________

Eye movement: ___________

Fontanel/window: ___________

Mood/affect: ___________

5. How did Tommy Douglas' neurologic assessment results change from early in his admission to the Pediatric Intensive Care Unit (PICU) on Monday to his admission to the telemetry unit on Wednesday? Document your findings below. (*Hint:* Go to the chart and review the Nurse's Notes and Physician's Notes.)

Monday

Wednesday

6. Number the following activities in order of priority, beginning with what you would assess first when examining a critically ill patient such as Tommy Douglas.

Activities	**Sequence**
_______ Check intravenous fluids and lines.	a. 1
_______ Perform a physical assessment.	b. 2
_______ Check ventilator settings.	c. 3
_______ Obtain vital signs.	d. 4

Head Injury Management

Reading Assignments:
Hockenberry: Wong's Essentials of Pediatric Nursing, 10th edition (Chapter 28)
Hockenberry: Wong's Nursing Care of Infants and Children, 10th edition (Chapter 33)

Patient: Tommy Douglas, Room 302

Objectives:

1. Analyze laboratory findings associated with acute head injury.
2. Participate in the care of a comatose child.
3. Review medications given to a child who has experienced a head injury.

Exercise 1

Virtual Hospital Activity

25 minutes

- Sign in to work at Pacific View Regional Hospital for Period of Care 1. (*Note:* If you are already in the virtual hospital from a previous exercise, click on **Leave the Floor** and then on **Restart the Program** to get to the sign-in window.)
- From the Patient List, select Tommy Douglas (Room 302).
- Click on **Go to Nurses' Station**.

1. Which of the following symptoms are commonly associated with diabetes insipidus (DI)? Select all that apply.

    _______ Excessive urination

    _______ Compensatory insatiable thirst

    _______ Dehydration

    _______ Electrolyte imbalance

    _______ Circulatory collapse

To complete questions 2 through 6, use the virtual hospital resources listed below. (*Remember:* To access the various resources, click on the icons on the toolbar at the top of your screen. When you have finished reviewing one resource and wish to move to another, always look for a navigational button in the lower right corner of your screen—for example, Return to Nurses' Station or Exit EPR.)

- Click on **Chart** and then on **302**.
- Click on and review the **Nurse's Notes** and **Laboratory Reports**.
- Click on **Return to Nurses' Station**.
- Click on **EPR** and then on **Login**. Choose **302** from the Patient drop-down menu and select various categories as needed.
- Click on **Exit EPR**.
- Click on **MAR** and then on tab **302** for Tommy Douglas' records.

2. List three symptoms of DI that are manifested in Tommy Douglas. (*Note:* Be specific; for example, "Tachycardia—HR greater than 120 bpm.")

3. What medication is being given to Tommy Douglas for the treatment of DI?

4. Complete the following table to describe the medication you identified in question 3. (*Hint:* Use the Drug Guide as needed.)

Drug	Action	Availability	Dose and Frequency for Children

5. What medications are used as part of Tommy Douglas' treatment to assist with blood pressure management? (*Hint:* Check the MAR and the Physician's Orders.)

6. Complete the following table to describe the medications you listed in question 5. (*Hint:* Use the Drug Guide as needed.)

Drug	Action	Availability	Dose and Frequency for Children

Acute Care Phase, Period of Care 1

Reading Assignments:
Hockenberry: Wong's Essentials of Pediatric Nursing, 10th edition (Chapters 19 and 27)
Hockenberry: Wong's Nursing Care of Infants and Children, 10th edition (Chapter 32)

Patient: Tommy Douglas, Room 302

Objectives:

1. Participate in the care of a comatose child.
2. Perform a neurologic assessment on a child who has experienced a head injury.
3. Review medications given to a child who has experienced a head injury.
4. Interpret assessment findings related to a child whose condition is unstable.

Exercise 1

Virtual Hospital Activity

35 minutes

- Sign in to work at Pacific View Regional Hospital for Period of Care 1. (*Note:* If you are already in the virtual hospital from a previous exercise, click on **Leave the Floor** and then on **Restart the Program** to get to the sign-in window.)
- From the Patient List, select Tommy Douglas (Room 302).
- Click on **Go to Nurses' Station**.
- Click on **Chart** at the top of the screen or click on the rack of charts in the center of the screen.
- Click on **302** for Tommy Douglas' chart.
- Click on **Physician's Orders** and review the orders written Wednesday morning.

1. List three orders written in Tommy Douglas' chart that are specific to the treatment of a child with a head injury.

- Click on **Return to Nurses' Station**.
- Click on **EPR** and then on **Login**.
- Choose **302** from the Patient drop-down menu and **Vital Signs** from the Category drop-down menu.

2. Evaluate Tommy Douglas' vital sign results Wednesday at 0700 (just before this shift). Are they normal for his age or his condition at the time?

Now take a current set of vital signs.

- Click on **Exit EPR** and then on **302** to go to Tommy Douglas' room.
- Inside the room, click on **Take Vital Signs**.

3. Record Tommy Douglas' current vital signs below.

4. What changes are reflected in the current vital sign findings that indicate a need for prompt intervention?

5. What should be done immediately to prevent further neurologic and systemic deterioration?

6. What should be given first to prevent systemic deterioration? Describe the initial intervention to correct the problem(s) identified in question 4.

- Click on **Chart** and then on **302**.
- Click on and review the **Physician's Orders**.

7. Which of the orders written at 0730 Wednesday has the most immediate effect on Tommy Douglas' blood pressure when implemented?

8. What additional physician's orders were written Wednesday morning at 0730 that are directly related to blood pressure stabilization?

- Click on **Return to Room 302** and then on **Medication Room** at the bottom of your screen.
- Click on **MAR** to determine what medications Tommy Douglas should receive at 0730. (*Note:* You may click on **Review MAR** at any time to verify the correct medication order. Remember to check the patient's name on the MAR to make sure you are viewing the correct record. You must click on the correct room number within the MAR.) Click on **Return to Medication Room** after reviewing the correct MAR.
- Click on **Unit Dosage** and then on drawer **302**.
- Click on the medication(s) you would like to administer. For each medication you select, click on **Put Medication on Tray**. When you are finished, click on **Close Drawer**.
- Click on **View Medication Room**.
- Click on **Automated System** and then on **Login**.
- Select the correct patient and drawer according to the medication you want to administer. (*Hint:* The automated system is for controlled substances only.) Then click on **Open Drawer**.
- Select the medication(s) you would like to administer, click on **Put Medication on Tray**, and then click on **Close Drawer**.
- Click on **View Medication Room**.
- Begin the preparation process by clicking on **Preparation** at the top of the screen or clicking on the tray on the counter on the left side of the Medication Room.
- From the list of medications you put on the tray, select the medication you wish to administer; then click on **Prepare**.
- Supply any information requested by the Preparation Wizard and then click on **Next**.
- Choose the correct patient to administer this medication to and click on **Finish**.
- Repeat the previous three steps until all medications that you want to administer are prepared.
- You can click on **Review Your Medications** and then on **Return to Medication Room** when ready.

Before you administer Tommy Douglas' medications, you must first check his existing intravenous (IV) lines and the fluids being administered.

- Click on **EPR** and then on **Login**.
- Select **302** from the Patient drop-down menu and **IV** from the Category drop-down menu.
- Review the data recorded on Wednesday at 0700.
- Now click on **Exit EPR**.
- Click on **Chart** and then on **302**.
- Select the **Physician's Orders** tab.
- Find the orders for Wednesday at 0600 and review to learn more about the fluids being infused through Tommy Douglas' IV lines.

9. Complete the following table to review the types of lines Tommy Douglas has and the fluids infusing through each line at 0700 on Wednesday.

Type of IV Line	Location of IV Line	Type of Fluid Infusing and Rationale for Using This IV Line
Central venous line		
Peripheral line		
Arterial line		

- Click on **Return to Medication Room**.
- Now click on **302** at the bottom of the screen to go to Tommy Douglas' room to administer his medication(s).
- Inside the room, click on **Patient Care** and then on **Medication Administration**.
- Next to the medication(s) you want to give, click on **Select** and choose **Administer** from the drop-down menu.
- Complete the Administration Wizard questions; then click on **Administer to Patient**.
- Specify **Yes** to document this to the MAR.
- Finally, click on **Finish**.

10. What vital signs would you assess to evaluate the effectiveness of implementing the intervention you identified in question 6?

- Click on **Patient Care** and then on **Nurse-Client Interactions**.
- Select and view the video titled **0800: Intervention—Stabilizing BP**. (*Note:* Check the virtual clock to see whether enough time has elapsed. You can use the fast-forward feature to advance the time by 2-minute intervals if the video is not yet available. Then click again on **Patient Care** and **Nurse-Client Interactions** to refresh the screen.)

The nurse informed Tommy Douglas' parents that she would be giving Tommy fluids to help stabilize his blood pressure. Let's jump forward in virtual time to see how effective this intervention was.

- Click on **Leave the Floor**.
- From the Floor Menu, select **Restart the Program**.
- Sign in for Period of Care 2.
- Choose Tommy Douglas as your patient; then click on **Go to Nurses' Station**.
- From the Nurses' Station, click on **EPR** and then on **Login**.
- Choose **302** from the Patient drop-down menu and **Vital Signs** from the Category drop-down menu.
- Use the left-pointing blue arrow at the bottom of the screen to move back to the data recorded on Wednesday at 0900.

11. What was Tommy Douglas' blood pressure at 0900 after the normal saline bolus was administered? Did his blood pressure improve as a result of this intervention?

Acute Care Phase, Period of Care 2

Reading Assignments:
   Hockenberry: Wong's Essentials of Pediatric Nursing, 10th edition (Chapters 17, 19, and 27)
   Hockenberry: Wong's Nursing Care of Infants and Children, 10th edition (Chapter 32)

Patient: Tommy Douglas, Room 302

Objectives:

1. Interpret physical assessment findings related to a child whose condition is unstable.
2. Evaluate laboratory data of the child with a head injury.
3. Observe interactions between health care providers and parents experiencing the loss of a child.

Exercise 1

Virtual Hospital Activity

20 minutes

- Sign in to work at Pacific View Regional Hospital for Period of Care 2. (*Note:* If you are already in the virtual hospital from a previous exercise, click on **Leave the Floor** and then on **Restart the Program** to get to the sign-in window.)
- From the Patient List, select Tommy Douglas (Room 302).
- Click on **Get Report.**
- Click on **Go to Nurses' Station**.
- Click on **302**.
- Inside Tommy Douglas' room, click on **Take Vital Signs**.

1. Document Tommy Douglas' current vital signs in the table below. Also, document these findings in the EPR. (*Hint:* If you need help with the steps for entering data in the EPR, see **A Quick Tour** in this workbook.)

Vital Sign	Findings
Temperature	
Systolic pressure	
Diastolic pressure	
Blood pressure mode of measurement	
Heart rate	
Respiratory rate	
Oxygen saturation (%)	

- Click on **Exit EPR**.
- In Tommy Douglas' room, review the Initial Observations.
- Next, click on **Patient Care** and then on **Physical Assessment**.
- Choose the various physical assessment areas and appropriate subcategories as needed to complete the table in question 2.

2. Record your findings from Tommy Douglas' physical assessment below and on the next page.

Assessment Area	Findings
General Appearance	
HEENT	
Pulmonary	
Cardiovascular	

Assessment	**Findings**
Gastrointestinal	
Genitourinary	
Musculoskeletal	
Neurologic	

- Now click on **Chart**.
- Click on **302** to access Tommy Douglas' chart.
- Review the **Physician's Orders** for 1100.
- Then click on **Laboratory Reports** and review the findings for Wednesday morning.

3. In the table below, record Tommy Douglas' CBC findings for Wednesday morning. Put an asterisk next to any abnormal findings.

Hematology Laboratory Test	Findings
Hemoglobin	
Hematocrit	
Platelets	

4. What has the physician ordered for Tommy Douglas at 1100?

5. What is the most likely rationale for this order, given Tommy Douglas' laboratory values at 1100?

6. What other medications are being infused at this same time?

- Still in the Laboratory Reports section, review Tommy Douglas' arterial blood gas values (ABGs) for 1100 on Wednesday.

7. Record Tommy Douglas' ABGs in the following table.

ABG Test	Findings—Wednesday 1100
PaO_2	
$PaCO_2$	
pH	
Bicarbonate	

8. Which type of acid-base imbalance is indicated by Tommy Douglas' 1100 ABG results?
   a. Metabolic alkalosis
   b. Respiratory alkalosis
   c. Respiratory acidosis
   d. Metabolic acidosis

- Review the **Physician's Orders** written for Tommy Douglas at 0820 on Wednesday.

9. What medication was ordered for Tommy Douglas at this time?

10. What is the most likely rationale for administering this medication to Tommy Douglas?

- Click on **Return to Room 302**.
- Click on **Patient Care** and then on **Nurse-Client Interactions**.
- Select and view the video titled **1115: The Family (Care) Conference**. (*Note:* Check the virtual clock to see whether enough time has elapsed. You can use the fast-forward feature to advance the time by 2-minute intervals if the video is not yet available. Then click again on **Patient Care** and **Nurse-Client Interactions** to refresh the screen.)
- After viewing the video, click on **Chart** and then on **302**.
- Review the **Physician's Notes** and **Consultations**.

11. What specific tests did the physicians review with Tommy Douglas' parents?

12. What specific findings on physical examination were listed in the consultation notes that concurred with brain death?

13. What is the caloric test?

- Click on **Return to Room 302**.
- Click on **Patient Care** and then on **Nurse-Client Interactions**.
- Select and view the video titled **1130: Decision—Organ Donation**. (*Note:* Check the virtual clock to see whether enough time has elapsed. You can use the fast-forward feature to advance the time by 2-minute intervals if the video is not yet available. Then click again on **Patient Care** and **Nurse-Client Interactions** to refresh the screen.)

14. What was discussed with Tommy Douglas' parents in the 1130 conference?

15. Who was present at the 1115 and 1130 family care conferences?

16. Why is a multidisciplinary team approach important for Tommy Douglas' family?

As a follow-up, let's check Tommy Douglas' 1300 repeat ABG results.

- Click on **Leave the Floor** and then on **Restart the Program**.
- Sign in to care for Tommy Douglas during Period of Care 3.
- Click on **Go to Nurses' Station** and then on **Chart**.
- Click on **302** and select **Laboratory Reports**.

17. Below, record Tommy's ABG results for Wednesday at 1300.

ABG Test	Findings—Wednesday 1300
PaO_2	
$PaCO_2$	
pH	
Bicarbonate	

6

Acute Care Phase, Period of Care 3

Reading Assignments:
Hockenberry: Wong's Essentials of Pediatric Nursing, 10th edition (Chapters 17, 19, and 27)
Hockenberry: Wong's Nursing Care of Infants and Children, 10th edition (Chapters 20 and 32)

Patient: Tommy Douglas, Room 302

Objectives:

1. Interpret physical assessment findings related to a child whose condition is unstable.
2. Evaluate laboratory data of the child with a head injury.
3. Observe interactions between health care providers and parents experiencing the loss of a child.
4. Describe the diagnostic evaluation necessary to confirm brain death in a child.

Exercise 1

Virtual Hospital Activity

30 minutes

- Sign in to work at Pacific View Regional Hospital for Period of Care 3. (*Note:* If you are already in the virtual hospital from a previous exercise, click on **Leave the Floor** and then on **Restart the Program** to get to the sign-in window.)
- From the Patient List, select Tommy Douglas (Room 302).
- Click on **Go to Nurses' Station**.
- Click on **302**; then click on **Take Vital Signs**.
- Document Tommy's 1500 vital signs results in the EPR. (*Hint:* If you need help entering data in the EPR, see **A Quick Tour** in this workbook.)
- When you have finished entering these data, click on **Exit EPR**.
- Now click on **Chart** and then on **302**.
- Click on **Physician's Orders**.

63

1. Why were new orders written at this time?

- Review Tommy Douglas' chart as needed to answer question 2.

2. In the left column below, list the tests used to establish brain death. In the right column, summarize the results of each of these tests for Tommy Douglas.

Diagnostic Test	Findings

- Click on **Return to Room 302**.
- Click on **Patient Care** and then on **Physical Assessment**.
- Click on **Head & Neck**.
- Click on **Neurologic** and complete a neurologic assessment on Tommy Douglas.
- Now click on **EPR** and then on **Login**.
- Select **302** from the Patient drop-down menu and **Neurologic** from the Category drop-down menu.
- Review the findings for Wednesday at 1400.

3. Based on your review of the EPR and the in-room neurologic assessment, record Tommy Douglas' neurologic findings for Wednesday at 1400 in the table below and on the next page.

Neurologic Assessment	Findings—Wednesday 1400
Glasgow Coma Scale: Eyes	
Glasgow Coma Scale: Verbal	
Glasgow Coma Scale: Motor	
Glasgow Coma Total Score	
Pupils Right: Size	
Pupils Right: Reaction	
Pupils Left: Size	

Neurologic Assessment	**Findings—Wednesday 1400**
Pupils Left: Reaction	
Cranial Nerves I-XII	
Orientation	
Speech	
Cognitive Perceptual	
Mental Status	
Sensation	

4. Are your physical examination findings consistent with the physician's and consultants' notes?

5. What is important for the nurse to know regarding organ donation when caring for a patient at the end of life?

- Click on **Exit EPR**.
- Once again, observe Tommy Douglas' vital signs on Wednesday 1400 by clicking on **Take Vital Signs**.

6. Record Tommy Douglas' current vital signs below.

Vital Sign	**Findings**
Temperature	
Systolic pressure	
Diastolic pressure	
Blood pressure mode of measurement	
Heart rate	
Respiratory rate	
Oxygen saturation (%)	

7. What continuing problem(s) do you anticipate for Tommy Douglas while waiting for organ procurement?

- Click on **Patient Care** and then on **Nurse-Client Interactions**.
- Select and view the video titled **1500: Nurse-Family Communication**. (*Note:* Check the virtual clock to see whether enough time has elapsed. You can use the fast-forward feature to advance the time by 2-minute intervals if the video is not yet available. Then click again on **Patient Care** and **Nurse-Client Interactions** to refresh the screen.)

8. What was reinforced by the nurse during this conversation?

9. Why was it important for the nurse in the video interaction to discuss ways for the family to remember Tommy Douglas?

- Click on **Patient Care** and then on **Nurse-Client Interactions**.
- Select and view the video titled **1515: The Grieving Family** to observe the specialist/family interaction. (*Note:* Check the virtual clock to see whether enough time has elapsed. You can use the fast-forward feature to advance the time by 2-minute intervals if the video is not yet available. Then click again on **Patient Care** and **Nurse-Client Interactions** to refresh the screen.)

10. Describe the role of a child life specialist and explain why this individual is an appropriate choice to meet with Tommy Douglas' siblings.

Providing Support for Families Experiencing the Loss of a Child

Reading Assignments:
Hockenberry: Wong's Essentials of Pediatric Nursing, 10th edition (Chapter 17)
Hockenberry: Wong's Nursing Care of Infants and Children, 10th edition (Chapter 20)

Patient: Tommy Douglas, Room 302

Objectives:

1. Provide nursing care for the child and family at the end of life.
2. Participate in the multidisciplinary care of the child at the end of life.

Exercise 1

Virtual Hospital Activity

45 minutes

- Sign in to work at Pacific View Regional Hospital for Period of Care 2. (*Note:* If you are already in the virtual hospital from a previous exercise, click on **Leave the Floor** and then on **Restart the Program** to get to the sign-in window.)
- From the Patient List, select Tommy Douglas (Room 302).
- Click on **Get Report** and read the clinical report.
- Click on **Go to Nurses' Station**.
- Click on **302** to go to Tommy Douglas' room.

1. Listed below are two patient problems appropriate for Tommy Douglas and his family at this time. Complete the table by identifying data that should be monitored and effective nursing interventions that should be used.

Patient Problem	Subjective and Objective Data (List at least 3 for each patient problem.)	Nursing Interventions (List at least 5 for each problem.)
Pain related to disease process		
Grieving related to impending loss of child		

- Click on **Patient Care** and then on **Nurse-Client Interactions**.
- Select and view the video titled **1115: The Family (Care) Conference**. (*Note:* Check the virtual clock to see whether enough time has elapsed. You can use the fast-forward feature to advance the time by 2-minute intervals if the video is not yet available. Then click again on **Patient Care** and **Nurse-Client Interactions** to refresh the screen.)

2. Complete the table below by answering the following question: What are important nursing care guidelines for supporting grieving families?

General Nursing Supports	At the Time of Death	After the Child Has Died

3. What are the ages of Tommy Douglas' siblings?

4. Based on the ages of Tommy Douglas' siblings, describe preschool and school-age children's typical reactions to death and identify possible interventions for support of Tommy's siblings.

Preschool children

School-age children

- Click on **Chart** and then on **302**.
- Click on **Consultations** and read the Social Services Consult and the Child Life Consult.

5. List at least four interventions found in the consultants' plans that provide an understanding of the health care roles of the following: chaplain, social worker, and child life specialist. Identify the interventions performed by each specific health care professional in this scenario.

6. What reactions do nurses commonly experience when facing the loss of a patient?

7. Identify at least three strategies that can assist nurses and other health care professionals to cope with the loss of a child in their care.

LESSON 8

Anorexia Nervosa: History and Physical Examination

Reading Assignments:
Hockenberry: Wong's Essentials of Pediatric Nursing, 10th edition (Chapters 16)
Hockenberry: Wong's Nursing Care of Infants and Children, 10th edition (Chapter 18)

Patient: Tiffany Sheldon, Room 305

Objectives:

1. Identify the early signs of anorexia nervosa.
2. Discuss the special care needs of the adolescent with anorexia nervosa.

Exercise 1

Virtual Hospital Activity

20 minutes

- Sign in to work at Pacific View Regional Hospital for Period of Care 1. (*Note:* If you are already in the virtual hospital from a previous exercise, click on **Leave the Floor** and then on **Restart the Program** to get to the sign-in window.)
- From the Patient List, select Tiffany Sheldon (Room 305).
- Click on **Go to Nurses' Station**.
- Click on **Chart** and then on **305**.
- Click on **Emergency Department** and review this report.

1. Describe Tiffany Sheldon's past illness history leading up to her Emergency Department visit.

2. List three treatment goals for patients with anorexia nervosa.

* While still in the chart, click on **Nursing Admission**.

3. Review the Nursing Admission and list three stressors found in Tiffany Sheldon's family.

* Now click on **Physician's Orders**.
* Note Tiffany Sheldon's medical diagnosis documented on the Physician's Orders for 0600 Wednesday.
* Click on **Return to Nurses' Station**.
* Click on **305** to enter Tiffany Sheldon's room.
* Click on **Patient Care** and then on **Physical Assessment**.
* Perform a focused physical assessment on Tiffany Sheldon.

4. List six findings from the physical assessment that relate to Tiffany Sheldon's diagnosis of malnutrition.

5. Based on the Emergency Department admission data and Tiffany Sheldon's past and present health history, list three appropriate patient problems with the etiology statement included.

6. What was Tiffany Sheldon's weight on admission to the Emergency Department?

7. What is Tiffany Sheldon's height? (*Hint:* Review the Nursing Admission in the chart.)

8. Using the CDC body mass index chart on the next page (Body mass index-for-age percentiles: Girls, 2 to 20 years), plot Tiffany Sheldon's body mass index (BMI) of 13.8 kg/m^2 according to her age: (weight in pounds/height in inches) / height in inches x 703. At what percentile is her BMI?

CDC Growth Charts: United States

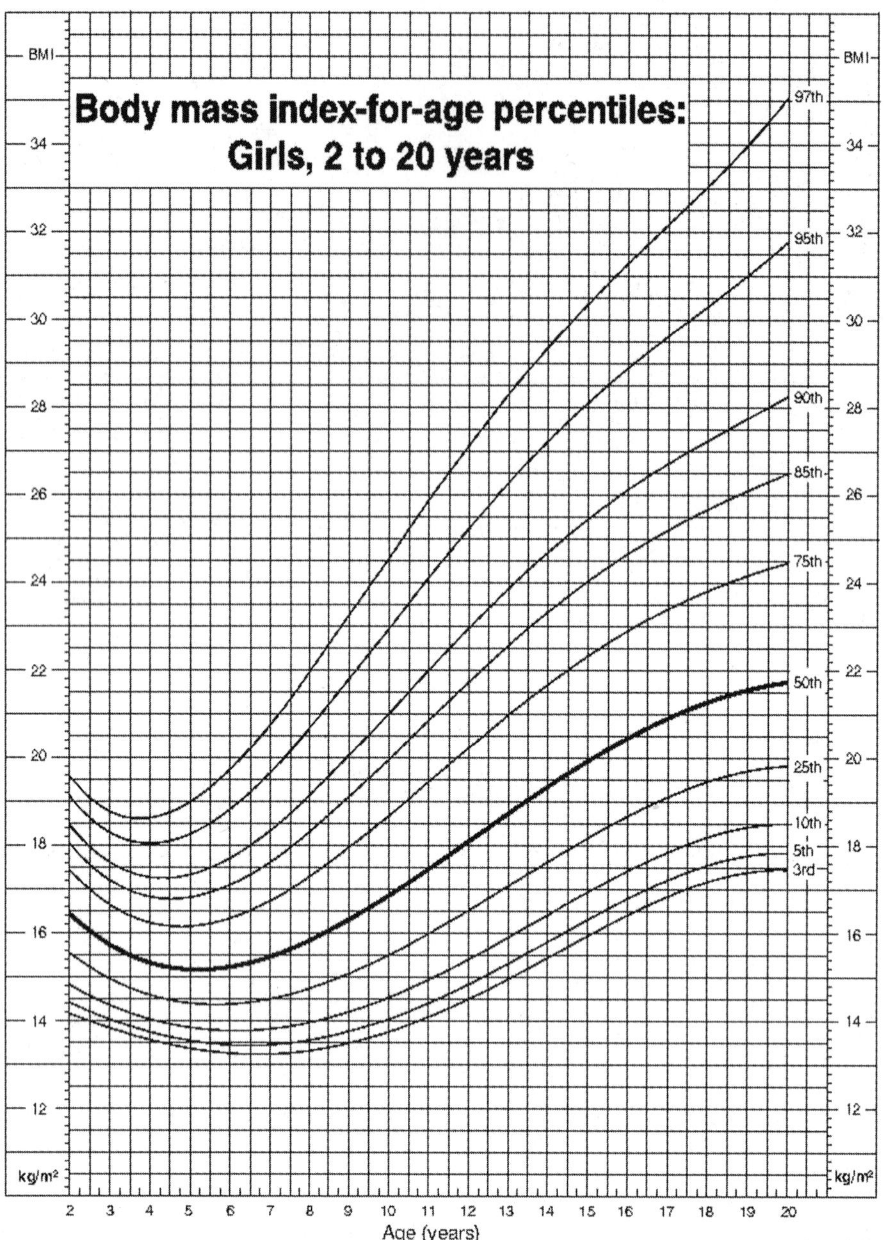

Published May 30, 2000.
SOURCE: Developed by the National Center for Health Statistics in collaboration with
the National Center for Chronic Disease Prevention and Health Promotion (2000).

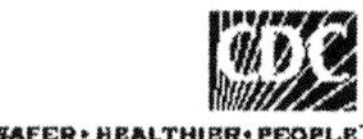

Pathophysiology of Anorexia Nervosa

Reading Assignments:
Hockenberry: Wong's Essentials of Pediatric Nursing, 10th edition (Chapter 16)
Hockenberry: Wong's Nursing Care of Infants and Children, 10th edition (Chapter 18)

Patient: Tiffany Sheldon, Room 305

Objectives:

1. Describe physical and behavioral characteristics of the adolescent with anorexia nervosa.
2. Identify family characteristics associated with the development of eating disorders in adolescents.

Exercise 1

Virtual Hospital Activity

15 minutes

- Sign in to work at Pacific View Regional Hospital for Period of Care 1. (*Note:* If you are already in the virtual hospital from a previous exercise, click on **Leave the Floor** and then on **Restart the Program** to get to the sign-in window.)
- From the Patient List, select Tiffany Sheldon (Room 305).
- Click on **Go to Nurses' Station**.
- Click on **Chart** and then on **305**.
- Click on **History and Physical**.

1. List three family characteristics that are associated with the development of an eating disorder such as anorexia nervosa.

2. What are some personality characteristics found in children with anorexia nervosa?
   a. Perfectionism, high achievement in academics, conformity, and conscientiousness
   b. Fearful, dependent, and controlling
   c. Goal-oriented, physically active, with erratic behaviors
   d. Independent, easy-going, poor academic performance

3. Which of the following is *not* a characteristic of anorexia nervosa?
   a. Pursuit of thinness
   b. Fear of fatness
   c. Disordered body perception
   d. Response to traumatic or personal life events
   e. Sequelae of infectious diseases

For questions 4 through 8, circle either True or False. For any statements you identify as false, provide a rationale for your decision.

4. Young people involved in competitive sports or activities such as ballet and gymnastics are also at risk for unsafe weight control practices and eating disorders such as anorexia nervosa.

   True / False

5. Bulimia nervosa is more common in females.

   True / False

6. An adolescent with anorexia may eventually develop bulimia.

   True / False

7. Patients with eating disorders such as anorexia nervosa usually do not have a psychiatric disorder or substance abuse problems.

True / False

8. The dominant aspects of anorexia nervosa are a persistent pursuit of thinness and a fear of fatness.

True / False

Anorexia Nervosa: Clinical Signs and Symptoms

Reading Assignments:
Hockenberry: Wong's Essentials of Pediatric Nursing, 10th edition (Chapters 4, 16, and 22)
Hockenberry: Wong's Nursing Care of Infants and Children, 10th edition (Chapters 4 and 24)

Patient: Tiffany Sheldon, Room 305

Objectives:

1. Identify the physical assessment characteristics of a child with anorexia nervosa.
2. Recognize potentially life-threatening physical assessment findings in the child with anorexia nervosa.
3. Identify diagnostic laboratory values indicative of dehydration.

Exercise 1

Virtual Hospital Activity

30 minutes

- Sign in to work at Pacific View Regional Hospital for Period of Care 1. (*Note:* If you are already in the virtual hospital from a previous exercise, click on **Leave the Floor** and then on **Restart the Program** to get to the sign-in window.)
- From the Patient List, select Tiffany Sheldon (Room 305).
- Click on **Go to Nurses' Station**.
- Click on **Chart** and then on **305**.
- Click on **Emergency Department** and review the record.

1. The Review of Systems in the Emergency Department revealed the findings in the right column below. Match each finding with the corresponding body system.

System	Finding
_____ Integumentary	a. Upper and lower extremity weakness
_____ Cardiovascular	b. 4-second capillary refill and 1+ pedal edema
_____ Genitourinary	c. Decreased skin turgor and dry skin
_____ Gastrointestinal	d. Constipation
_____ Neuromuscular	e. Decreased urine output

2. List the clinical findings of Tiffany Sheldon's physical examination documented by the nurse and physician in the Emergency Department.

3. Identify initial clinical findings in the Emergency Department record that require immediate attention.

4. Describe the most likely cause of the findings you identified in question 3, as well as the significance of the findings.

- Click on **Return to Nurses' Station**.
- Click on **305** to go to Tiffany Sheldon's room.
- Click on **Patient Care** and then on **Nurse-Client Interactions**.
- Select and view the video titled **0730: Initial Assessment**. (*Note:* Check the virtual clock to see whether enough time has elapsed. You can use the fast-forward feature to advance the time by 2-minute intervals if the video is not yet available. Then click again on **Patient Care** and **Nurse-Client Interactions** to refresh the screen.)

5. In the video, what assessment does the nurse perform related to Tiffany Sheldon's cardiovascular status?

6. What else does the nurse ask Tiffany Sheldon in the video that relates to the cardiovascular assessment?

- Click on **Chart** and then **305**.
- Select **Laboratory Reports**.
- Review the findings documented in the Emergency Department on Wednesday at 0530.

7. Below, record Tiffany Sheldon's laboratory results obtained in the Emergency Department. For each test, provide the normal range of values for a child Tiffany Sheldon's age (14).

Test	Tiffany Sheldon's Result	Normal Range
Glucose		
Sodium		
Potassium		
Chloride		
Creatinine—serum		
BUN		
Calcium—serum, total		
Protein—serum		
Albumin—serum		

8. Tiffany Sheldon's initial specific gravity is 1.035. What does specific gravity measure? What is the significance of this clinical finding in relation to Tiffany Sheldon's clinical status?

- Now click on and review the initial **Physician's Orders**.

9. Tiffany Sheldon is being treated for dehydration. What laboratory tests are ordered to assess and monitor the status of her dehydration?
   a. Albumin, protein, and alkaline phosphatase
   b. HCG urinalysis and specific gravity
   c. Glucose, phosphorus, calcium, and magnesium
   d. BUN, creatinine, Chem 7, and specific gravity

10. What is the purpose of obtaining a urine HCG on Tiffany Sheldon?

11. Tiffany Sheldon has been diagnosed with malnutrition. What laboratory tests are ordered to assess and monitor her malnutrition?
   a. Serum VDRL, specific gravity, and alkaline phosphatase
   b. Protein, albumin, glucose, and alkaline phosphatase
   c. Protein, calcium, ALT, and AST
   d. Chem 7, protein, and BUN

12. Tiffany Sheldon has been diagnosed with bradycardia. Which of these laboratory tests are ordered to assess and monitor her cardiac function?
   a. BUN, creatinine, protein, and glucose
   b. Chem 7, VDRL, specific gravity, and alkaline phosphatase
   c. Chem 7, phosphorus, calcium, and magnesium
   d. ALT, AST, urine specific gravity, and protein

- Next, click on **Nursing Admission** and review.

13. For which of the following risks was Tiffany Sheldon assessed on admission? Select all that apply.

   ______ Risk for infection

   ______ Risk for hypertension

   ______ Risk for falls

   ______ Risk for impaired tissue integrity

14. What is the underlying cause of these assessed risks?
   a. Poor nutrition, electrolyte imbalance, and muscle wasting
   b. Poor nutrition, depression, and too much exercise
   c. Amenorrhea, electrolyte imbalance, and depression
   d. Muscle wasting, depression, and too much exercise

15. What is the best explanation for the finding of lanugo in Tiffany Sheldon's physical examination?
    a. Hair follicles are starved of the appropriate nutrition needed to produce healthy hair.
    b. It is the result of cold intolerance in an attempt to warm the body.
    c. It is secondary to cardiac insufficiency.
    d. All of the above explain Tiffany Sheldon's findings.

16. For which of the following reasons should rapid weight gain be avoided in patients with anorexia nervosa? Select all that apply.

    _______ It has been associated with refeeding syndrome.

    _______ Cardiovascular, neurologic, and hematologic complications can arise when nutritional replacement occurs too rapidly.

    _______ Patients with anorexia nervosa are fearful of gaining weight.

    _______ Patients with anorexia nervosa have a distorted body image.

17. Urinary tract problems are frequent in patients with anorexia nervosa, including the presence of ketones and proteins in the urine. What is the most likely cause of these findings?
    a. Low body temperature
    b. Fat and protein breakdown
    c. Decreased cardiac output

18. Tiffany Sheldon complains of problems with constipation. This finding is related to which of the following? Select all that apply.

    _______ Delayed gastric emptying

    _______ Decreased fluid intake

    _______ Muscle wasting

    _______ Reduced intestinal motility

19. Which of the following physical symptoms of anorexia nervosa does Tiffany Sheldon *not* have? Select all that apply.

    _______ Lowered body temperature

    _______ Bradycardia

    _______ Decreased blood pressure

    _______ Cold intolerance

    _______ Headaches

    _______ Vomiting

    _______ Secondary amenorrhea

20. What best explains the finding of edema on Tiffany Sheldon's admission?

21. List two laboratory values from question 7 that are helpful in evaluating the malnourished patient.

Management of Anorexia Nervosa

Reading Assignments:
Hockenberry: Wong's Essentials of Pediatric Nursing, 10th edition (Chapter 16)
Hockenberry: Wong's Nursing Care of Infants and Children, 10th edition (Chapters 18 and 29)

Patient: Tiffany Sheldon, Room 305

Objectives:

1. Describe the contents and identify the goal of the behavioral therapy plan/contract.
2. List priority goals in the treatment of anorexia nervosa.
3. Describe the role of the multidisciplinary health care team in the management of anorexia nervosa.

Exercise 1

Writing Activity

5 minutes

1. Which of the following are goals of treatment for anorexia nervosa? Select all that apply.

_______ Reinstitution of normal nutrition or reversal of the severe state of malnutrition

_______ Resolution of disturbed patterns of family interaction

_______ Individual psychotherapy to correct deficits and distortions of psychologic functioning

_______ Neurologic assessment to evaluate for physical therapy

2. Which of the following are goals of behavioral therapy with the patient who has anorexia nervosa? Select all that apply.

_____ To allow the patient to have some individual control and responsibility toward recovery

_____ To gradually reverse the malnutrition

_____ To establish a structured environment in which team members provide consistency and continuity

_____ To provide support for the patient's efforts and give positive feedback for accomplishments made in normalizing eating habits

Exercise 2

Virtual Hospital Activity

25 minutes

Note: For this exercise, you will need to observe and consider four video interactions in two different periods of care before answering questions. Therefore you may wish to review questions 1 through 8 before signing in and then take notes while you view the videos.

- Sign in to work at Pacific View Regional Hospital for Period of Care 2. (*Note:* If you are already in the virtual hospital from a previous exercise, click on **Leave the Floor** and then on **Restart the Program** to get to the sign-in window.)
- From the Patient List, select Tiffany Sheldon (Room 305).
- Click on **Go to Nurses' Station**.
- Click on **305** to go to Tiffany Sheldon's room.

For the first video:

- Click on **Patient Care** and then on **Nurse-Client Interactions**.
- Select and view the video titled **1115: Managing Anorexia Nervosa**. (*Note:* Check the virtual clock to see whether enough time has elapsed. You can use the fast-forward feature to advance the time by 2-minute intervals if the video is not yet available. Then click again on **Patient Care** and **Nurse-Client Interactions** to refresh the screen.)

For the second video:

- Click again on **Patient Care** and then on **Nurse-Client Interactions**.
- View the video titled **1130: Monitoring Compliance**.
- When you have finished viewing this video, click on **Leave the Floor**.
- At the Floor Menu, select **Restart the Program**.

For the third video:

- Sign in again to care for Tiffany Sheldon, this time for Period of Care 3.
- Click on **Go to Nurses' Station** and then on **305**.
- Again, click on **Patient Care** and then on **Nurse-Client Interactions**.
- Select and view the video titled **1500: Relapse—Contributing Factors**.

For the fourth video:

- Click again on **Patient Care** and then on **Nurse-Client Interactions**.
- Select and view the video titled **1530: Facilitating Success**.
- After watching the fourth video interaction, complete questions 1 through 8.

1. List four things that Tiffany Sheldon has agreed to in her behavioral therapy plan/contract.

2. What statement does Tiffany Sheldon make during the video interactions that may lead you to believe she has concerns about her weight and caloric intake?

3. Why do you think the nurse asked Tiffany Sheldon's mother to allow her to speak to Tiffany alone?

4. What behavioral modification plans are implemented and discussed with Tiffany Sheldon? What are these plans specifically designed to monitor?

5. What purpose would monitoring Tiffany Sheldon in the bathroom serve in regard to food intake?

6. The precise cause of anorexia nervosa is unknown; however, recommendations for management have suggested that treatment is best managed by an interdisciplinary team. Ideally, which of the following should be included on the team? Select all that apply.

_____ Dietitians

_____ Physicians and nurses

_____ Counselors

_____ Psychologists or psychiatrists

For questions 7 through 11, circle either True or False. For any statement you identify as false, provide a rationale for your decision.

7. The self-damaging behaviors of anorexia nervosa are a result of the patient's distorted body image and self-awareness, feelings of self-doubt, ineffectiveness, helplessness, and lack of control.

   True / False

8. Individual team members can make alterations to the behavioral modification plan based on their individual interactions with the patient who has anorexia nervosa.

   True / False

9. If the patient views the behavioral therapy approach as coercive and becomes depressed by the approach, it is possible that weight gain may not be sustained outside the hospital.

   True / False

10. Pharmacotherapy has been extremely successful in the treatment of anorexia nervosa in adolescent patients.

    True / False

11. Patients with bulimia tend to be more likely to maintain rigid control than do patients with anorexia nervosa.

    True / False

Nursing Care of the Child with Anorexia Nervosa

Reading Assignments:
Hockenberry: Wong's Essentials of Pediatric Nursing, 10th edition (Chapter 16)
Hockenberry: Wong's Nursing Care of Infants and Children, 10th edition (Chapter 18)

Patient: Tiffany Sheldon, Room 305

Objectives:

1. Describe the contents and identify the goal of the behavioral therapy plan/contract.
2. Describe the psychologic implications of food intake in relation to perceived body image in the adolescent with anorexia nervosa.
3. Discuss the role of cognitive behavioral therapy in patients with anorexia nervosa.

Exercise 1

Virtual Hospital Activity

20 minutes

- Sign in to work at Pacific View Regional Hospital for Period of Care 2. (*Note:* If you are already in the virtual hospital from a previous exercise, click on **Leave the Floor** and then on **Restart the Program** to get to the sign-in window.)
- From the Patient List, select Tiffany Sheldon (Room 305).
- Click on **Go to Nurses' Station**.
- Click on **Chart** and then on **305**.
- Click on **Consultations**.
- Review the Nutrition Consult at 1100.
- Click on **Return to Nurses' Station** and then on **305** to go to Tiffany Sheldon's room.
- Click on **Patient Care** and then on **Nurse-Client Interactions**.
- Select and view the video titled **1115: Managing Anorexia Nervosa**. (*Note:* Check the virtual clock to see whether enough time has elapsed. You can use the fast-forward feature to advance the time by 2-minute intervals if the video is not yet available. Then click again on **Patient Care** and **Nurse-Client Interactions** to refresh the screen.)
- Next, select and view the video titled **1130: Monitoring Compliance**.

93

1. The dietitian has been working with Tiffany Sheldon and is aware of her history. In the 1115 video interaction, what is the purpose of the visit with Tiffany Sheldon? Select all that apply.

   _______   To develop the eating contract

   _______   To get Tiffany Sheldon's agreement about the eating contract

   _______   To assess Tiffany Sheldon's current nutritional status

   _______   To present Tiffany Sheldon with a menu to help in selection of a diet

2. What concern does Tiffany Sheldon express during the video interaction with the dietitian?
   a. She is concerned about when she will be discharged from the hospital.
   b. She is concerned that she will not be able to consume all the calories in the contract.
   c. She is concerned that the diet will make her more constipated.
   d. She is concerned that the diet will make her gain weight too quickly.

3. What are possible barriers to Tiffany Sheldon being successful in negotiating the eating contract?
   a. Difficulty thinking clearly because of her poor nutritional status
   b. Inability to find hospital foods that are acceptable to her
   c. Unwillingness to remain in the hospital
   d. Concern about missing school

4. The dietitian is working with a treatment team to help monitor progress. What is the most important medical risk involved in developing a nutritional plan for Tiffany Sheldon?
   a. Possible physical injury from too much exercise
   b. Worsening constipation from increasing the diet
   c. Complications of refeeding syndrome, leading to severe metabolic abnormalities and cardiac complications

- Click on **Chart**.
- Click on **305** for Tiffany Sheldon's chart.
- Click on **Consultations** and review the Psychiatric Consult at 1500 on Wednesday.

5. What are the main goals of cognitive behavioral therapy in the adolescent with anorexia nervosa? Select all that apply.

   _______   To promote the correction of metabolic abnormalities

   _______   To ensure a quick return to normal body weight

   _______   To develop a therapeutic alliance to permit open discussion of the patient's feelings and help develop more appropriate ways to communicate and cope

   _______   To provide individual cognitive therapy to deal with environmental, familial, and personal conditions that may lead to anorexia nervosa

6. Identify three underlying issues that the psychiatrist identifies as contributing factors in Tiffany Sheldon's illness.

For questions 7 through 10, circle either True or False. For any statement you identify as false, provide a rationale for your decision.

7. An additional purpose for cognitive behavioral therapy in anorexia nervosa is to help the patient develop a locus of control in order to express herself in acceptable ways.

   True / False

8. Sports that emphasize leanness or sports in which weight class is prerequisite to participation have been associated with a higher incidence of eating disorders.

   True / False

9. It is important for the patient to understand that the team is in control of the contract and that the patient must obey all parts of the contract without question.

   True / False

10. It is important to provide family members with support to help them deal with the pressures of managing a patient with anorexia nervosa.

    True / False

LESSON 13

Emergent Nursing Care of the Child with Meningitis

Reading Assignments:
Hockenberry: Wong's Essentials of Pediatric Nursing, 10th edition (Chapters 4 and 27)
Hockenberry: Wong's Nursing Care of Infants and Children, 10th edition (Chapters 4 and 32)

Patient: Stephanie Brown, Room 304

Objectives:

1. Analyze laboratory findings associated with childhood meningitis.
2. Differentiate between bacterial and aseptic meningitis.
3. Describe the components of a neurologic assessment for a child who is diagnosed with meningitis.
4. Describe the pathophysiology of meningitis.

Exercise 1

Writing Activity

5 minutes

1. Match the following terms with the corresponding characteristics.

Term	**Characteristic**
_____ Meningitis	a. Viral inflammation of the meninges
_____ Mode of meningitis transmission	b. Greatest morbidity between birth and 4 years
_____ Bacterial meningitis	c. Vascular dissemination of mucosal organisms frequently from the nasopharyngeal site
_____ Predisposition to meningitis	d. Pyogenic inflammation of the meninges
_____ Aseptic meningitis	e. Inflammation of the membranes covering the brain and spinal cord

2. What are common clinical manifestations of meningitis in children and adolescents?

Exercise 2

Virtual Hospital Activity

45 minutes

- Sign in to work at Pacific View Regional Hospital for Period of Care 1. (*Note:* If you are already in the virtual hospital from a previous exercise, click on **Leave the Floor** and then on **Restart the Program** to get to the sign-in window.)
- From the Patient List, select Stephanie Brown (Room 304).
- Click on **Go to Nurses' Station**.
- Click on **304** to go to Stephanie Brown's room.
- Click on **Patient Care** and then on **Physical Assessment**.
- Click on **Head & Neck**.
- Click on **Neurologic** and view the assessment.

1. State the physiologic basis for Stephanie Brown's headache.

- Click on **Chart**.
- Click on **304** to view Stephanie Brown's Chart.
- Click on **Emergency Department** and review.
- Then click on and read the **Nurse's Notes** and **Physician's Notes**.

2. List the clinical manifestations of meningitis exhibited by Stephanie Brown in the Emergency Department.

- Click on and read the **History and Physical** section of Stephanie Brown's chart.

3. Describe the Glasgow Coma Scale and list the three-part assessment of the coma scale.

- Click on **Laboratory Reports**. Review the findings recorded in the Emergency Department on Monday at 0100.

4. Below, list the abnormal findings you noted for Stephanie Brown in the Laboratory Reports. For each abnormal finding, give the normal range of results. Finally, what does each finding indicate?

Laboratory Test	Abnormal Results	Normal Range	Indications

- Now click on **Diagnostic Reports** and review the summary of Stephanie Brown's lumbar puncture.

5. When a child has suspected meningitis, cerebral spinal fluid (CSF) pressure can be measured during the lumbar puncture with a manometer. What is Stephanie Brown's CSF pressure? What is the significance of these results in relation to Stephanie Brown's condition? (*Hint:* The normal range for a child her age is 60-100 mm H_2O.)

6. Below, list each of the CSF results from Stephanie Brown's lumbar puncture on Monday. For each finding, give the normal range of results and identify what each finding indicates.

CSF (Lumbar)	Results	Normal Range	Indications

7. What is the rationale for placing Stephanie Brown in respiratory isolation?

- Click on **Physician's Orders** and review.

8. What medication is ordered for Stephanie Brown for a high temperature?

9. What is the rationale for administering this medication per rectum (PR) in the Emergency Department at 0100 on Monday?

10. What is the rationale for having the head of Stephanie Brown's bed elevated 45 degrees?

11. Describe the standard isolation technique for a child with meningitis in an acute care center. (*Note:* You may describe the standard practice in an institution where you work as staff member or student.)

12. What is the physiologic basis for giving Stephanie Brown a normal saline bolus in the Emergency Department? (*Hint:* See the Systems Review section of the Emergency Department record in the chart.)

- Click on **Return to Room 304**.
- Click on **MAR** and review Stephanie Brown's records.

13. An intravenous infusion is started immediately in a child with suspected meningitis to administer IV fluids and:
    a. antiepileptic drugs.
    b. steroid drugs.
    c. blood products.
    d. antimicrobial drugs.

14. Give a rationale for your answer to question 13.

Now let's go to the Medication Room and prepare to administer all of the 0730 and 0800 medications ordered for Stephanie Brown.

- First, click on **Return to Room 304**.
- Next, click on **Medication Room**.
- Click on **MAR** to determine what medications Stephanie Brown should receive for 0730 and 0800. You may review the MAR at any time to verify the correct medication order. (*Hint:* Remember to look at the patient name on the MAR to make sure you have the correct record. You must click on the tab with Stephanie Brown's room number within the MAR.) Click on **Return to Medication Room** after reviewing the correct MAR.
- Click on **Unit Dosage** and then on drawer **304**.
- Select the medications you would like to administer. For each medication you select, click on **Put Medication on Tray**. When you are finished, click on **Close Drawer**.
- Click on **View Medication Room**.
- Now click on **Automated System** and **Login**.
- Select the correct patient and drawer according to the medication you want to administer. (*Hint:* This automated system is for controlled substances only.) Then click on **Open Drawer**.
- Select the medication you would like to administer, click on **Put Medication on Tray**, and then click on **Close Drawer**.
- Click on **View Medication Room**.
- Click on **Preparation** and select the medication to administer.
- Click on **Prepare** and wait for the Preparation Wizard to appear. If the Wizard requests information, provide your answer(s) and then click on **Next**.
- Choose the correct patient and then click on **Finish**.
- Repeat the previous three steps until all medications that you want to administer are prepared.
- You can click on **Review Your Medications** and then click on **Return to Medication Room** when ready. Once you are back in the Medication Room, go directly to Stephanie Brown's room by clicking on **304** at the bottom of the screen.

- In Stephanie Brown's room, administer the medications, using the six rights of medication administration. After you have collected the appropriate assessment data and are ready for administration, click on **Patient Care** and then on **Medication Administration**. Verify that the correct patient and medication(s) appear in the left-hand window. Then click on the down arrow next to Select. From the drop-down menu, select **Administer** and complete the Administration Wizard by providing any information requested. When the Wizard stops asking for information, click on **Administer to Patient**. Specify **Yes** when asked whether this administration should be recorded in the MAR. Finally, click on **Finish**. Complete these steps for each medication you wish to administer.

15. In the mock MAR form below, document the medications you administered.

Medication/Dose	2300-0700	0700-1500	1500-2300

16. Stephanie Brown is receiving maintenance IV fluids with strict intake and output to prevent what severe complication?

- To answer questions 17 through 19, you will need to consult the virtual hospital Drug Guide.
- To access the Drug Guide, click on the **Drug** icon in the lower left corner of your screen. When the Drug Guide opens, use the Search bar or scroll through the alphabetic list of drugs at the top of the screen; select **vancomycin**.

17. Provide the rationale for the intravenous administration of this drug (versus oral administration).

18. Briefly describe the procedure for administering vancomycin intravenously to a child Stephanie Brown's age. Include the correct dilution, if required.

19. List three serious side effects for which the nurse should be vigilant during and after the administration of this medication.

Now let's see how you did administering Stephanie's medications.

- Click on **Leave the Floor** at the bottom of your screen. From the Floor Menu, select **Look at Your Preceptor's Evaluation**. Then click on **Medication Scorecard**.
- Review the scorecard to see whether or not you correctly administered the appropriate medication(s). If not, why do you think you were incorrect? According to Table C in this scorecard, what resources should have been used and what important assessments should have been completed before administering the medication(s)? Did you use these resources and perform these assessments correctly?
- Print a copy of the Medication Scorecard for your instructor to evaluate.

Nursing Care of the Hospitalized Child

Reading Assignments:
Hockenberry: Wong's Essentials of Pediatric Nursing, 10th edition (Chapters 22 and 27)
Hockenberry: Wong's Nursing Care of Infants and Children, 10th edition (Chapters 1 and 32)

Patient: Stephanie Brown, Room 304

Objectives:

1. Describe the nursing care of the child with meningitis and constipation.
2. Identify the rationale for auditory testing in the child with meningitis.

Exercise 1

Virtual Hospital Activity

45 minutes

- Sign in to work at Pacific View Regional Hospital for Period of Care 2. (*Note:* If you are already in the virtual hospital from a previous exercise, click on **Leave the Floor** and then on **Restart the Program** to get to the sign-in window.)
- From the Patient List, select Stephanie Brown (Room 304).
- Click on **Go to Nurses' Station**.
- Click on **Chart** and then on **304**.
- Click on **Emergency Department** and review the record.
- Click on and review the **Physician's Orders** and **Physician's Notes** for Wednesday at 0900.
- Click on **Return to Nurses' Station**.
- Click on **304** to go to Stephanie Brown's room.
- Click on **Patient Care** and then on **Nurse-Client Interactions**.
- Select and view the video titled **1120: Preventing Spread of Disease**. (*Note:* Check the virtual clock to see whether enough time has elapsed. You can use the fast-forward feature to advance the time by 2-minute intervals if the video is not yet available. Then click again on **Patient Care** and **Nurse-Client Interactions** to refresh the screen.)

1. What might explain why the physician decreased Stephanie Brown's IV rate to 10 mL/hr?

2. How did Stephanie Brown's nurse explain the basis for the respiratory isolation?

3. Based on your earlier review of the Physician's Notes, what was the physician's most likely rationale for discontinuing the respiratory isolation and vancomycin for Stephanie Brown?

- Still in Stephanie Brown's room, click on **Clinical Alerts** and review.

4. What does the Clinical Alert say regarding Stephanie's abdominal assessment?

5. When did Stephanie Brown have her last bowel movement?

- Return to Stephanie Brown's chart and review the **Physician's Notes** to answer question 6.

6. Compare the Monday and Wednesday notes in regard to the Kernig sign, Brudzinski sign, and nuchal rigidity results for Stephanie Brown. Record any changes below.

- Click on **Return to Room 304**.
- Click on **MAR** and review Stephanie Brown's medication orders.

7. Are there further indications for performing an audiogram on this patient (besides the diagnosis of meningitis)?

- Click on **Return to Room 304**.
- Click on **Chart** and then on **304**.
- Click on **Physician's Orders** and review the orders for 1100 on Wednesday.

8. What medication is ordered for Stephanie Brown at this time?

- Click on **Return to Room 304**.
- Click on the **Drug** icon in the lower left corner of your screen. Locate and review the information for the drug ordered for Stephanie Brown.

9. Complete the following table for the drug you identified in question 8. Relate your answers specifically to Stephanie Brown's need for the medication.

Name of Medication	Classification	Action	Dosage	Frequency	Route

- Click on **Return to Room 304**.
- Click on **Medication Room**.
- Prepare the medication you identified in question 8.
- When you have finished the steps of the Preparation Wizard, click on **Return to Medication Room** and then on **304** to go to Stephanie Brown's room.
- Administer the medication, using the six rights of medication administration.
- After you have collected the appropriate assessment data and are ready for administration, click on **Patient Care** and then on **Medication Administration**. Verify that the correct patient and medication(s) appear in the left-hand window. Then click the down arrow next to Select. From the drop-down menu, select **Administer** and complete the Administration Wizard by providing any information requested. When the Wizard stops asking for information, click on **Administer to Patient**. Specify **Yes** when asked whether this administration should be recorded in the MAR. Finally, click on **Finish**.

10. In the mock MAR form below, document the medication you just administered to Stephanie Brown. Indicate the time you gave it in the correct column.

Medication/Dose	2300-0700	0700-1500	1500-2300

Now let's see how you did!

- Click on **Leave the Floor** at the bottom of your screen. From the Floor Menu, select **Look at Your Preceptor's Evaluation**. Then click on **Medication Scorecard**.
- Review the scorecard to see whether or not you correctly administered the appropriate medication. If not, why do you think you were incorrect? According to Table C in this scorecard, what resources should be used and what important assessments should be completed before administering the medication(s)? Did you utilize these resources and perform these assessments correctly?
- Print a copy of the Medication Scorecard for your instructor to evaluate.

Next, let's evaluate Stephanie's vital signs, especially her pain level.

- Click on **Return to Evaluations** and then on **Return to Menu**.
- Click on **Restart the Program** and sign in for Period of Care 2.
- From the Patient List, select Stephanie Brown (Room 304).
- Click on **Go to Nurses' Station**.
- Click on **EPR** and then on **Login**.
- Select **304** from the Patient drop-down menu and **Vital Signs** from the Category drop-down menu.

11. Compare Stephanie Brown's blood pressure and pain scale rating on Wednesday 0700 with her BP and pain rating on Wednesday at 1100.

12. a. Using the FACES pain rating scale below, which face matches Stephanie Brown's description of her headache recorded on Wednesday at 1100?

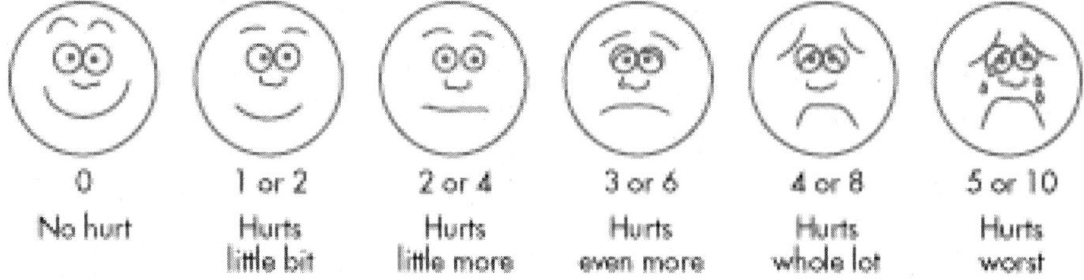

   b. Identify the three scales used in the FACES system.

- Click on **Exit EPR**.
- Click on **Chart** and then on **304**.
- Once again, review the **Physician's Orders** for Stephanie Brown.

13. What is ordered that can be administered to alleviate Stephanie Brown's headache?

- Click on **Return to Nurses' Station**.
- Now click on the **Drug** icon in the lower left corner of your screen.

14. Using the Drug Guide as your reference, complete the following table for the medication you identified in question 13.

Name of Medication	Classification	Action	Dosage	Frequency	Route

- Click on **Return to Nurses' Station**.
- Click on **Chart** and then on **304**.
- Review the **Nurse's Notes** for Tuesday at 2300 and Wednesday at 0600.

15. Based on your assessment of Stephanie Brown at this time, what route would be appropriate for administering the medication you identified in question 13? State your rationale for choosing this route.

16. Briefly describe the indication(s) for administering baclofen to the child with cerebral palsy. (*Hint:* Use the Drug Guide.)

- Still in the chart, click on **Consultations** and review the Audiology Consult.
- Click on **Return to Nurses' Station** and then on **304**.
- Click on **Patient Care** and then on **Nurse–Client Interactions**.
- Select and view the video titled **1145: Teaching—Disease Sequelae**. (*Note:* Check the virtual clock to see whether enough time has elapsed. You can use the fast-forward feature to advance the time by 2-minute intervals if the video is not yet available. Then click again on **Patient Care** and **Nurse-Client Interactions** to refresh the screen.)

17. Explain the basis for obtaining the audiogram for Stephanie Brown. State the results of the audiogram.

Nursing Care of the Hospitalized Child with Cerebral Palsy

Reading Assignments:
  Hockenberry: Wong's Essentials of Pediatric Nursing, 10th edition (Chapters 19 and 30)
  Hockenberry: Wong's Nursing Care of Infants and Children, 10th edition (Chapters 5, 26, and 35)

Patient: Stephanie Brown, Room 304

Objectives:

1. Discuss the special needs of a child with cerebral palsy (CP).
2. Describe the issues involved in discharge planning and home care of the child with CP.
3. Identify measures to decrease anxiety in a child and family with meningitis.

Exercise 1

Virtual Hospital Activity

50 minutes

- Sign in to work at Pacific View Regional Hospital for Period of Care 3. (*Note:* If you are already in the virtual hospital from a previous exercise, click on **Leave the Floor** and then on **Restart the Program** to get to the sign-in window.)
- From the Patient List, select Stephanie Brown (Room 304).
- Click on **Go to Nurses' Station**.
- Click on **304** to go to the patient's room.
- Click on **Patient Care** and then on **Nurse-Client Interactions**.
- Select and view the video titled **1500: Assessment—IV Site**. (*Note:* Check the virtual clock to see whether enough time has elapsed. You can use the fast-forward feature to advance the time by 2-minute intervals if the video is not yet available. Then click again on **Patient Care** and **Nurse-Client Interactions** to refresh the screen.)

1. How did the nurse describe the IV site in the video? What are the implications of her findings?

- Click on **Patient Care** and then on **Nurse-Client Interactions**.
- Now select and view the video titled **1510: Nurse-Patient Communication**. (*Note:* Check the virtual clock to see whether enough time has elapsed. You can use the fast-forward feature to advance the time by 2-minute intervals if the video is not yet available. Then click again on **Patient Care** and **Nurse-Client Interactions** to refresh the screen.)

2. The nurse in the video states that she will apply EMLA cream before restarting Stephanie Brown's IV. What is the purpose of doing this?

Let's take a virtual leap in time to see whether the EMLA cream was actually applied.

- First, click on **Leave the Floor** and then on **Restart the Program**.
- Sign in to work with Stephanie Brown for Period of Care 4.
- Click on **MAR** and then on tab **304**. (*Remember:* You are not able to visit patients or administer medications during Period of Care 4. You are able to review patient records only.)
- Review Stephanie Brown's MAR for Wednesday at 1900.

3. At what time was the EMLA cream administered? Why should the nurse wait 60 minutes after EMLA is applied to the skin before the IV is restarted?

Now, let's return to Period of Care 3 to continue your care for Stephanie Brown.

- Once again, click on **Leave the Floor** and then on **Restart the Program**.
- Sign in to work with Stephanie Brown for Period of Care 3.
- Click on **Go to Nurses' Station**.
- Click on **Chart** and then on **304**.
- Click on **History and Physical** and review.
- Click on **Nursing Admission** and review.

4. List the predisposing maternal and perinatal factors in Stephanie Brown's history that may have contributed to the development of CP.

* Click on **Consultations** and read the PT/OT consult.

5. State the findings of the PT/OT consult.

6. What specific therapy is recommended for Stephanie Brown by the physical therapist based on the findings during the consult?

7. What is an ankle-foot orthosis (AFO)? When did Stephanie Brown start wearing an AFO? State the purpose of her AFO.

* Click on **Nurse's Notes**.
* Review the Nurse's Notes from the Emergency Department admission through Wednesday.

8. What specific request does Stephanie Brown's mother make of the social worker? (*Hint:* Read the note on Tuesday at 1500.)

9. Describe activities that can help Stephanie Brown's mother cope with the anxiety associated with her daughter's hospitalization and life-threatening illness.

10. Describe age-appropriate activities that can help Stephanie Brown cope with the anxiety associated with hospitalization and respiratory isolation.

11. What recommendations could you give Stephanie Brown's mother to promote Stephanie's daily bowel movement?

- Click on **Return to Nurses' Station**.
- Click on **304** to go to Stephanie Brown's room.
- Click on **Patient Care** and then on **Nurse-Client Interactions**.
- Select and view the video titled **1530: Preventive Measures**. (*Note:* Check the virtual clock to see whether enough time has elapsed. You can use the fast-forward feature to advance the time by 2-minute intervals if the video is not yet available. Then click again on **Patient Care** and **Nurse-Client Interactions** to refresh the screen.)

12. What specific recommendation does the physical therapist make to Stephanie Brown's mother on the consult note and during the video?

LESSON 16

Care of the Infant with Respiratory Distress

Reading Assignments:
Hockenberry: Wong's Essentials of Pediatric Nursing, 10th edition (Chapters 4, 20, 21, and 22)
Hockenberry: Wong's Nursing Care of Infants and Children, 10th edition
      (Chapters 11, 22, 24, 27, and 28)

Patient: Carrie Richards, Room 303

Objectives:

1. Recognize signs of acute respiratory distress in an infant.
2. Describe interventions to treat respiratory distress in an infant.
3. Describe the nursing care of an infant with respiratory syncytial virus (RSV) and bronchiolitis.

Exercise 1

Writing Activity

30 minutes

1. What is respiratory syncytial virus (RSV)? Briefly describe the characteristic progression of this illness in infants. Also identify any associated clinical manifestations.

2. How is this illness transmitted?

3. Describe the steps that can be taken to reduce or prevent the transmission of this illness.

4. List four priority nursing interventions for an infant with RSV.

5. What medication may be given as prophylactic treatment for RSV in high-risk patients? Who should receive the medication, and when should this medication be administered? How is the medication given?

Exercise 2

Virtual Hospital Activity

50 minutes

- Sign in to work at Pacific View Regional Hospital for Period of Care 1. (*Note:* If you are already in the virtual hospital from a previous exercise, click on **Leave the Floor** and then on **Restart the Program** to get to the sign-in window.)
- From the Patient List, select Carrie Richards (Room 303).
- Click on **Go to Nurses' Station**.
- Click on **Chart** and then on **303** for Carrie Richards' chart.
- Click on **Emergency Department** and review the record.

1. What are Carrie Richards' vital signs on admission to the Emergency Department (ED) at 1630? Put an asterisk next to any findings that are out of normal range for a child her age.

2. Briefly describe the findings for Carrie Richards recorded in the ED Systems Review and in the ED Nurse's Note at 1800. Put an asterisk next to any findings that are abnormal for a child Carrie Richards' age.

3. List the five cardinal clinical signs of respiratory distress in an infant.

- Still in the Emergency Department section of the chart, compare the findings in the ED Nurse's Notes at 1800 and 1900.

4. What clinical signs documented by the nurse indicate a change in Carrie Richards' respiratory status at 1900?

5. What specific intervention is performed to improve Carrie Richards' oxygenation status?

6. What medication is administered to Carrie Richards to improve her respiratory status in the ED?

7. Describe the intended effect of this medication in a child with bronchiolitis/RSV who is wheezing and has a lower airway infection.

8. Describe how this medication is administered in an infant Carrie Richards' age. What is the rationale for this method of administration?

9. List two side effects of this medication.

10. Identify priority assessments that need to be performed after the nebulizer treatment is given.

11. What is the primary medical diagnosis listed for Carrie Richards?

12. List two patient problems for Carrie Richards based on your review of her status in the ED.

13. In the 1800 ED nurse's notes, an important clue is given in relation to the severity of Carrie Richards' status. What might lead you to conclude that her condition is poor? (*Hint:* Consider her age and developmental status.)

- Still in Carrie Richards' chart, click on **Laboratory Reports**.

14. Below, fill in Carrie Richards' laboratory values recorded in the ED at 1800 on Tuesday.

Chemistry	Results	Arterial Blood Gas	Results
Glucose		pH	
Sodium (serum)		PaO_2	
Potassium		$PaCO_2$	
Chloride		Oxygen sat	
CO_2			
Creatinine			
BUN			
Calcium			

Urinalysis	Results	Hematology	Results
Color		WBC	
Clarity		RBC	
Glucose		Hgb	
Bilirubin		Hct	
Blood		Platelets	
Spec gravity		Differential	
pH		Segs	
Protein		Bands	
Ketones		Lymphocytes	
WBC		Monocytes	
		Eosinophils	
		Basophils	

15. Which laboratory values in the table in question 14 are out of normal range for a child Carrie Richards' age?

- Click on **Emergency Department**. Once again, review the ED Nurse's Notes for 1900 on Tuesday.

16. How is Carrie Richards' respiratory status described? What interventions other than the nebulized medication administration and oxygen were performed to improve her respiratory status? State the rationale for the intervention performed.

17. List the clinical signs, physical assessment findings, and any laboratory values that provide a basis for determining Carrie Richards' hydration status on admission to the ED.

18. Describe the intervention(s) used to hydrate Carrie Richards in the ED.

19. List two reasons Carrie Richards is *not* a candidate for oral hydration in the ED.

20. Describe important assessment data that should be documented regarding Carrie Richards' IV site.

Care of the Hospitalized Infant

Reading Assignments:
Hockenberry: Wong's Essentials of Pediatric Nursing, 10th edition (Chapters 4, 20, and 21)
Hockenberry: Wong's Nursing Care of Infants and Children, 10th edition
(Chapters 4, 6, 23, 24, and 28)

Patient: Carrie Richards, Room 303

Objectives:

1. Identify physical assessment findings in the infant with respiratory distress.
2. Describe the nursing care of an infant with respiratory syncytial virus (RSV) and bronchiolitis.

Exercise 1

Virtual Hospital Activity

20 minutes

- Sign in to work at Pacific View Regional Hospital for Period of Care 1. (*Note:* If you are already in the virtual hospital from a previous exercise, click on **Leave the Floor** and then on **Restart the Program** to get to the sign-in window.)
- From the Patient List, select Carrie Richards (Room 303).
- Click on **Get Report**.
- Click on **Go to Nurses' Station**.
- Click on **Chart** and then on **303**.
- Click on and review the **Emergency Department** records.
- Click on and review **History and Physical**.
- Click on and review the **Nursing Admission** and the **Physician's Orders** for Tuesday 1700 and 2300.

1. Briefly summarize Carrie Richards' health history since birth.

2. Is Carrie Richards' immunization status current? If not, list the immunization(s) she should receive as soon as possible.

- Before leaving the chart, record Carrie Richards' physical assessment findings on admission in the middle column of the table in question 3. (*Hint:* You can find these in the Emergency Department Record.)
- After recording these findings, click on **Return to Nurses' Station**.
- Click on **303** to go to Carrie Richards' room.
- Click on **Patient Care** and then on **Physical Assessment**.
- Perform a focused assessment by clicking on the body system categories (yellow buttons) and subcategories (green buttons) as needed to complete question 3.

3. Record your findings from the physical assessment (her current in-room findings) in the far-right column below. Then compare these current findings with those obtained on admission to the Emergency Department (those you found in her chart).

Findings	Admission 1700 Tuesday	Current Findings
Respiratory effort		
Breath sounds		
Adventitious lung sounds		
Sensory/activity level		
Capillary refill		
Pulses		
Supplemental oxygen		

- Still in Carrie Richards' room, click on **Patient Care** and then on **Nurse-Client Interactions**.
- Select and view the video titled **0730: Patient Assessment**. (*Note:* Check the virtual clock to see whether enough time has elapsed. You can use the fast-forward feature to advance the time by 2-minute intervals if the video is not yet available. Then click again on **Patient Care** and **Nurse-Client Interactions** to refresh the screen.)

4. How does the nurse assess Carrie Richards' respiratory status in the video?

5. Carrie Richards is 3½ months old. At this age, breathing is primarily:
   a. abdominal.
   b. diaphragmatic.

- Click on **Take Vital Signs**.

6. Record Carrie Richards' vital sign results below.

7. Based on Carrie Richards' current physical assessment findings and vital signs, what conclusion might be drawn about her respiratory status and general health at this time?

- Click on **EPR** and then on **Login**.
- Select **303** from the Patient drop-down menu.
- Choose various categories as needed to record the vital signs and physical assessment finding you gathered in Carrie Richards' room. Be sure to include respiratory findings and IV status. (*Note:* The EPR may be printed for instructor evaluation.)

Exercise 2

Virtual Hospital Activity

45 minutes

- Sign in to work at Pacific View Regional Hospital for Period of Care 3. (*Note:* If you are already in the virtual hospital from a previous exercise, click on **Leave the Floor** and then on **Restart the Program** to get to the sign-in window.)
- From the Patient List, select Carrie Richards (Room 303).
- Click on **Go to Nurses' Station**.
- Click on **Chart** and then on **303**.
- Review the **Nurse's Notes**.
- Click on **Return to Nurses' Station**.
- Click on **EPR** and then on **Login**.
- Select **303** from the Patient drop-down menu and **Respiratory** from the Category drop-down menu.

1. Summarize Carrie Richards' respiratory status at 1300 on Wednesday based on the 1240 Nurse's Notes and 1215 respiratory assessment data in the EPR.

- Still in the EPR, change the category to **Vital Signs**.

2. What is Carrie Richards' body temperature at 1445?

- Click on **Exit EPR**.
- Click on **MAR** and then on tab **303**.

3. What medication does Carrie Richards have ordered for fever or irritability?

Now let's go to the Medication Room and prepare to administer all of the 1500 medications ordered for Carrie Richards.

- First, click on **Return to Nurses' Station**.
- Next, click on **Medication Room**.

- Click on **MAR** to determine what medications Carrie Richards should receive for 1500. You may review the MAR at any time to verify the correct medication order. (*Hint:* Remember to look at the patient name on the MAR to make sure you have the correct record. You must click on the tab with Carrie's room number within the MAR.) Click on **Return to Medication Room** after reviewing the correct MAR.

- Click on **Unit Dosage** and then on drawer **303**.

- Select the medications you would like to administer. For each medication you select, click on **Put Medication on Tray**. When you are finished, click on **Close Drawer**.

- Click on **View Medication Room**.

- Now click on **Automated System** and then on **Login**.

- Select the correct patient and drawer according to the medication you want to administer. (*Hint:* This automated system is for controlled substances only.) Then click on **Open Drawer**.

- Select the medication you would like to administer, click on **Put Medication on Tray**, and then click on **Close Drawer**.

- Click on **View Medication Room**.

- Click on **Preparation** and select the medication to administer.

- Click on **Prepare** and wait for the Preparation Wizard to appear. If the Wizard requests information, provide your answer(s), and then click on **Next**.

- Choose the correct patient and then click on **Finish**.

- Repeat the previous three steps until all medications that you want to administer are prepared.

- You can click on **Review Your Medications** and then on **Return to Medication Room** when ready. Once you are back in the Medication Room, go directly to Carrie Richards' room by clicking on **303** at the bottom of the screen.

- In Carrie Richards' room, administer the medications, using the six rights of medication administration. After you have collected the appropriate assessment data and are ready for administration, click on **Patient Care** and then on **Medication Administration**. Verify that the correct patient and medication(s) appear in the left-hand window. Then click the down arrow next to Select. From the drop-down menu, select **Administer** and complete the Administration Wizard by providing any information requested. When the Wizard stops asking for information, click on **Administer to Patient**. Specify **Yes** when asked whether this administration should be recorded in the MAR. Finally, click on **Finish**. Complete these steps for each medication you wish to administer.

Now let's see how you did!

- Click on **Leave the Floor** at the bottom of your screen. From the Floor Menu, select **Look at Your Preceptor's Evaluation**. Then click on **Medication Scorecard**.

- Review the scorecard to see whether or not you correctly administered the appropriate medication(s). If not, why do you think you were incorrect? According to Table C in this scorecard, what resources should be used and what important assessments should be completed before administering the medication(s)? Did you use these resources and perform these assessments correctly?

- Print a copy of the Medication Scorecard for your instructor to evaluate.

4. How does the nurse evaluate pain or discomfort in an infant Carrie Richards' age?

- Click on **Return to Evaluations** and then on **Return to Menu**.
- Click on **Restart the Program** and sign in for Period of Care 3.
- From the Patient List, select Carrie Richards (Room 303).
- Click on **Go to Nurses' Station** and then on **303**.
- In Carrie Richards' room, click on **Patient Care** and then on **Nurse-Client Interactions**.
- Select and view the video titled **1500: Teaching—Oral Medication**. (*Note:* Check the virtual clock to see whether enough time has elapsed. You can use the fast-forward feature to advance the time by 2-minute intervals if the video is not yet available. Then click again on **Patient Care** and **Nurse-Client Interactions** to refresh the screen.)

5. How does the nurse teach Carrie Richards' mother (Brenda) to administer Carrie's oral medication?

6. What statement(s) does Brenda make about Carrie's eating habits in the last few days before admission?

7. What interrelated factors should the nurse consider when an infant has a compromising respiratory illness such as RSV/bronchiolitis and the infant's food intake is decreased?

8. What are the implications of these findings for an infant in relation to hydration status and present illness?

9. What concerns does Carrie Richards' mother express about her daughter's nutritional status?

10. How does the nurse address Brenda's concerns about Carrie's nutritional status?

11. An infant's illness and hospitalization may represent a significant stressor for a single mother and her infant. What can the nursing staff do to minimize Brenda's anxiety about her child's hospitalization?

Nutritional Assessment and Discharge Planning

Reading Assignments:
Hockenberry: Wong's Essentials of Pediatric Nursing, 10th edition (Chapters 10 and 19)
Hockenberry: Wong's Nursing Care of Infants and Children, 10th edition (Chapters 10, 11, and 22)

Patient: Carrie Richards, Room 303

Objectives:

1. Assess the nutritional status of the infant with suspected growth failure (failure to thrive).
2. Describe the nursing care of the infant with growth failure (failure to thrive), including family interventions for home care and management.

Exercise 1

Virtual Hospital Activity

20 minutes

- Sign in to work at Pacific View Regional Hospital for Period of Care 1. (*Note:* If you are already in the virtual hospital from a previous exercise, click on **Leave the Floor** and then on **Restart the Program** to get to the sign-in window.)
- From the Patient List, select Carrie Richards (Room 303).
- Click on **Get Report**.
- Click on **Go to Nurses' Station**.
- Click on **Chart** and then on **303**.
- Click on and review the **Emergency Department** report and the **History and Physical**.
- Click on and review the **Nursing Admission** and the **Physician's Notes** for Tuesday at 1700 and 2300.

1. What was Carrie Richards' weight on admission to the Emergency Department?

2. What observations were made regarding the appearance of Carrie Richards' body size in the Emergency Department?

3. What additional observations were made by the staff that address Carrie Richards' overall nutritional status?

4. What is Carrie Richards' secondary medical diagnosis in the Emergency Department?

5. What is the rationale for weighing Carrie Richards again on Wednesday morning at 0755?

6. Review the WHO/CDC growth chart on the following page (Birth to 36 months: Girls—Length-for-Age and Weight-for-Age Percentiles). Plot Carrie Richards' admission weight and length on the chart.

   Carrie Richards is just below the _______ percentile for weight-for-age and at the

   _______ percentile for length-for-age at $3\frac{1}{2}$ months.

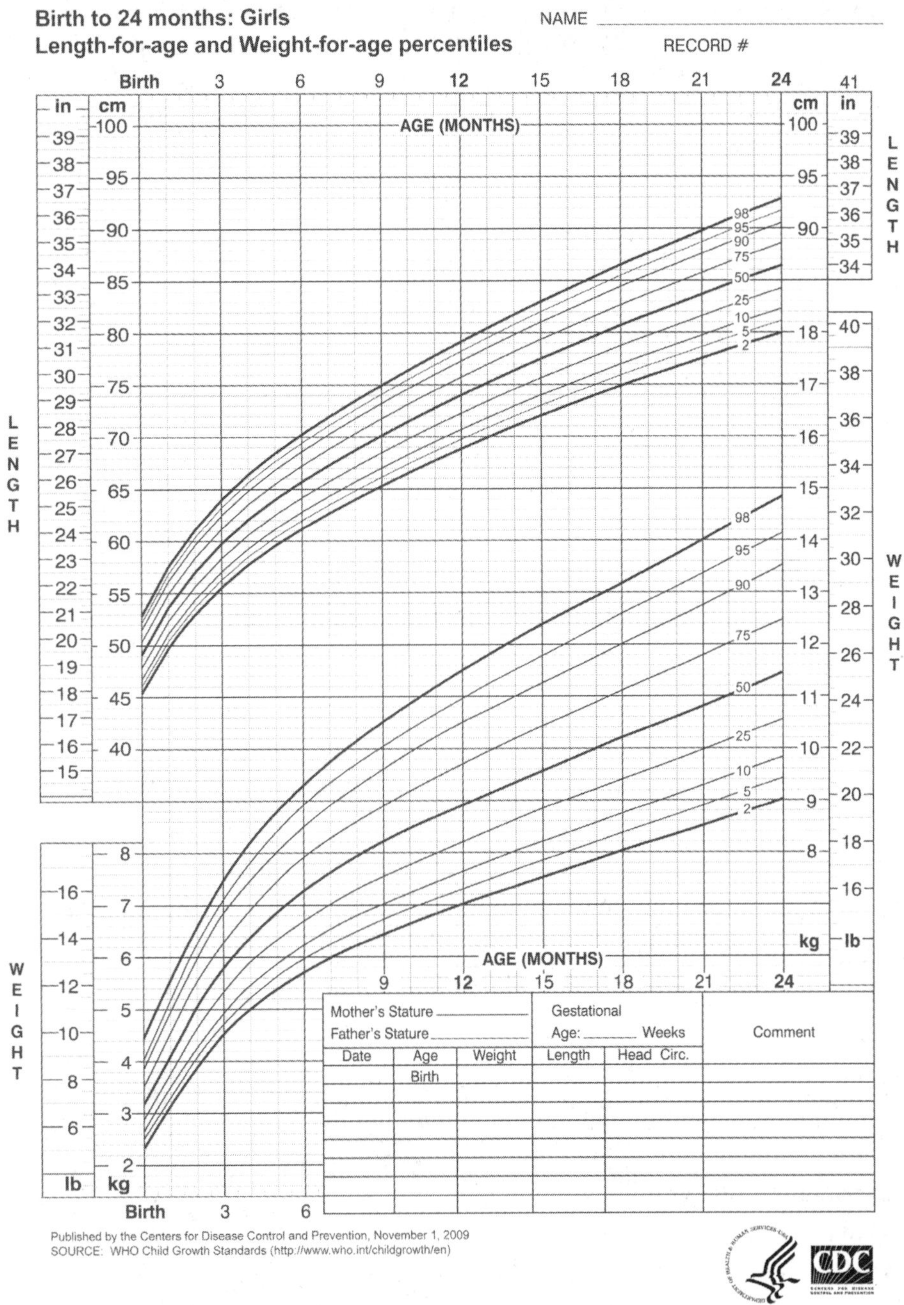

7. What is the significance of these findings for an infant Carrie Richards' age?

- Once again, review Carrie Richards' **History and Physical** and **Nursing Admission** in the chart.

8. In the dietary history there is significant information regarding Carrie Richards' feedings. What does the mother say she has been feeding her daughter? (Include amounts and frequency as applicable.)

9. What is the significance of the information you listed in question 8?

10. What is the rationale for the addition of rice cereal to a nighttime bottle?

11. Is the practice of putting an infant to sleep with a nighttime bottle recommended? Why?

- Click on **Return to Nurses' Station**.
- Click on **303** to go to Carrie Richards' room.
- Click on **Patient Care** and then on **Nurse-Client Interactions**.
- Select and view the video titled **0800: Assessment—Fact Finding**. (*Note:* Check the virtual clock to see whether enough time has elapsed. You can use the fast-forward feature to advance the time by 2-minute intervals if the video is not yet available. Then click again on **Patient Care** and **Nurse-Client Interactions** to refresh the screen.)

12. What assessment does the nurse in the video tell the mother she will make to assess Carrie Richards' ability to tolerate feedings in relation to her condition?

13. What additional observations might the nurse make at the time of feeding?

14. How is the diagnosis of growth failure established?

Exercise 2

Virtual Hospital Activity

15 minutes

- Sign in to work at Pacific View Regional Hospital for Period of Care 2. (*Note:* If you are already in the virtual hospital from a previous exercise, click on **Leave the Floor** and then on **Restart the Program** to get to the sign-in window.)
- From the Patient List, select Carrie Richards (Room 303).
- Click on **Go to Nurses' Station**.
- Click on **Chart** and then on **303**.
- Click on **Consultations** and read the Dietary/Nutrition Consult.

1. What does the dietitian report regarding Carrie Richards' nutritional status?

2. According to the consult findings, what additional information is discovered about how Carrie Richards is fed that has a significant impact on the number of calories she has been receiving?

3. How might the nurse assess the report that Carrie Richards spits up frequently after feedings?

- Now click on **Nurse's Notes** and review the notes for Wednesday at 1240, 1425, and 1500.

4. Briefly summarize Carrie Richards' feeding pattern since the acute phase of respiratory stress has resolved and her breathing has improved.

5. What is MCT oil? Why is it added to Carrie Richards' formula?

6. Write two measurable outcomes for weight gain and caloric (formula) intake for Carrie Richards for the next few days. Include specifics on how these outcomes will be measured.

7. Some interventions have been addressed dealing with Carrie Richards' growth failure. Identify additional nursing interventions that would be appropriate to implement in the hospital setting to help the mother care for Carrie.

Exercise 3

Virtual Hospital Activity

10 minutes

- Sign in to work at Pacific View Regional Hospital for Period of Care 3. (*Note:* If you are already in the virtual hospital from a previous exercise, click on **Leave the Floor** and then on **Restart the Program** to get to the sign-in window.)
- From the Patient List, select Carrie Richards (Room 303).
- Click on **Go to Nurses' Station**.
- Click on **Chart** and then on **303**.
- Click on **Consultations** and review the Social Service Consult at 1430 on Wednesday.
- While in the chart, also review the **Nursing Admission** and the **History and Physical**.

1. Describe Carrie Richards' mother's family situation, marital status, sources of economic support, and any other factors that may influence her ability to care for herself and her daughter.

2. Devise a plan for postdischarge follow-up for Carrie Richards and her mother. Consider the mother's lack of transportation, the need for close medical follow-up to assess Carrie's progress over the next few weeks, and the limited family resources. Set up the plan for Carrie's discharge on Thursday morning and evaluate the feasibility of the plan, assuming that her respiratory status continues to improve as it has since admission Tuesday evening.

LESSON 19

Emergent Care of the Child with Diabetic Ketoacidosis

Reading Assignments:

Hockenberry: Wong's Essentials of Pediatric Nursing, 10th edition (Chapters 14, 19, 22, and 28)
Hockenberry: Wong's Nursing Care of Infants and Children, 10th edition
(Chapters 15, 22, 24, and 33)

Patient: George Gonzalez, Room 301

Objectives:

1. Recognize the clinical manifestations of diabetic ketoacidosis (DKA) in a child with type 1 diabetes mellitus (DM).
2. Describe the pathophysiology of DKA in a child with type 1 DM.
3. Describe the nursing care of the child with DKA.
4. Identify significant diagnostic laboratory tests in the management of type 1 DM.

Exercise 1

Virtual Hospital Activity

30 minutes

- Sign in to work at Pacific View Regional Hospital for Period of Care 1. (*Note:* If you are already in the virtual hospital from a previous exercise, click on **Leave the Floor** and then on **Restart the Program** to get to the sign-in window.)
- From the Patient List, select George Gonzalez (Room 301).
- Click on **Go to Nurses' Station**.
- Click on **Chart** and then on **301** for George Gonzalez's record.
- Click on **Emergency Department**.

139

1. What were George Gonzalez's primary and secondary medical diagnoses on admission to the Emergency Department?

2. List three clinical manifestations of DKA.

3. What is the significance of vomiting in a child who has DKA?

4. List altered neurologic signs the nurse should be alert for in a child with DKA.

- Click on **Laboratory Reports** and review the initial blood work drawn in the Emergency Department at 1730 on Tuesday.

5. What was George Gonzalez's blood glucose result on admission?

6. List the normal blood glucose values for a child George Gonzalez's age.

7. Complete the table below with George Gonzalez's laboratory values and normal parameters.

Laboratory Tests	George Gonzalez's Values	Normal Parameters
Sodium (serum)		
Potassium (serum)		
BUN		
Creatinine		
CO_2 (serum)		
Urine ketones		
Urine glucose		
Urine specific gravity		
Arterial pH		
$PaCO_2$		
PaO_2		
WBC		
Hgb		
Hct		
Platelets		
RBC		

8. Based on George Gonzalez's laboratory values in questions 5 and 7, is the diagnosis of DKA supported at this time?

9. Identify the initial intervention performed in the Emergency Department to rehydrate George.

10. What nursing observations are particularly important for a child with DKA who is receiving intravenous fluids?

11. What is the significance of monitoring cardiac function in a child with DKA?

- Click on **Physician's Orders** and review the orders for George Gonzalez in the Emergency Department at 1730.

12. What medication is ordered?

13. What is the preferred method for administering insulin to a patient with DKA?

14. How is George Gonzalez's insulin administered in the Emergency Department at 1730?

15. What is the rationale for admitting the child with DKA to an intensive care unit?

16. What are Kussmaul respirations?

17. What is the significance of Kussmaul respirations in ketoacidosis?

Care of the Hospitalized Child with Type 1 Diabetes Mellitus

Reading Assignments:
Hockenberry: Wong's Essentials of Pediatric Nursing, 10th edition (Chapter 28)
Hockenberry: Wong's Nursing Care of Infants and Children, 10th edition (Chapter 33)

Patient: George Gonzalez, Room 301

Objectives:

1. Differentiate between type 1 and type 2 diabetes mellitus (DM).
2. Differentiate between the types of insulin used in the child with type 1 DM.
3. Identify specific learning and emotional needs of the preadolescent with a chronic illness.

Exercise 1

Virtual Hospital Activity

45 minutes

- Sign in to work at Pacific View Regional Hospital for Period of Care 1. (*Note:* If you are already in the virtual hospital from a previous exercise, click on **Leave the Floor** and then on **Restart the Program** to get to the sign-in window.)
- From the Patient List, select George Gonzalez (Room 301).
- Click on **Go to Nurses' Station**.
- Click on **Chart** and then on **301** for George's record.
- Click on and review the **History and Physical** and **Nursing Admission** sections of the chart.

1. List the three Ps that are cardinal signs associated with type 1 DM. Briefly explain the significance of each term.

145

2. In the table below, identify the main differences between type 1 and type 2 DM.

Characteristics	Type 1 DM	Type 2 DM
Type of onset		
Sex ratio		
Presenting symptoms		
Nutritional status		
Serum insulin (natural)		
Chronic complications		
Ketoacidosis		
Therapy Used		
Insulin		
Oral agents		
Diet only		

3. Diabetes mellitus may mimic other illnesses and may be overlooked. What are some of the accompanying signs and symptoms that may cause one to overlook DM?

4. What was George Gonzalez's $HgbA_{1c}$ (glycosylated hemoglobin) on admission to the Emergency Department?

5. The primary goals of DM treatment are to maintain glucose levels of __________ mg/dL and a glycosylated hemoglobin ($HgbA_{1c}$) less than _____%.

6. What is the significance of the $HgbA_{1c}$ in a person with DM in relation to compliance with the medical regimen and long-term complications?

- Click on **Return to Nurses' Station** and then on **301**.
- Click on **Patient Care** and then on **Nurse-Client Interactions**.
- Select and view the video titled **0730: Supervision—Glucose Testing**. (*Note:* Check the virtual clock to see whether enough time has elapsed. You can use the fast-forward feature to advance the time by 2-minute intervals if the video is not yet available. Then click again on **Patient Care** and **Nurse-Client Interactions** to refresh the screen.)

7. What does George Gonzalez say about checking his glucose at home?

8. What skill does the nurse ask George Gonzalez to perform during this interaction?

9. What is the significance of the nurse observing George Gonzalez check his glucose instead of checking it for him?

10. What was George Gonzalez's fingerstick blood glucose at 0745 on Wednesday?

- Click on **Chart** and then on **301**.
- Click on **Physician's Orders** and review the orders written at 2200 on Tuesday.
- Click on **Return to Room 301**.
- Now click on **MAR** and review George Gonzalez's MAR for Wednesday morning.

11. What intervention should occur once George Gonzalez has checked his blood glucose level before breakfast?

12. In addition to monitoring his glucose levels, what additional psychomotor skill should George Gonzalez be expected to perform in relation to diabetic management?

13. List the doses and types of insulin George Gonzalez is to administer before his breakfast.

14. What step should be taken to prevent hypoglycemia when a rapid-acting insulin is administered?

Insulin is now available in a number of premixed forms that make administration easier. These forms include the insulin pump and insulin pen. The insulin pump and pen may not be available to all children because of cost and skill level. George Gonzalez may be a candidate for administering insulin with an insulin pen.

15. Briefly describe the advantages of an insulin pen for a person George Gonzalez's age.

16. What is the rationale for using both types of insulin throughout the day?

17. Briefly describe how you would draw up the following: lispro 6 units and NPH 12 units. Be specific about the order in which you would complete these steps. (*Remember:* Clear insulin, then cloudy insulin.)

18. Regular insulin is:
    a. best administered at least 30 minutes after a meal.
    b. best administered at least 30 minutes before a meal.
    c. best administered immediately after a meal.
    d. best administered immediately before a meal.

- Click on **Return to Room 301**.
- Click on **Patient Care** and then on **Nurse-Client Interactions**.
- Select and view the video titled **0745: Self-Administering Insulin**. (*Note:* Check the virtual clock to see whether enough time has elapsed. You can use the fast-forward feature to advance the time by 2-minute intervals if the video is not yet available. Then click again on **Patient Care** and **Nurse-Client Interactions** to refresh the screen.)

19. In the video, what specific task does the nurse ask George Gonzalez to perform?

20. In this video interaction, how does the nurse evaluate George Gonzalez's understanding of his diabetes?

21. Based on your observation of George Gonzalez's actions in this video and his responses to the nurse about his condition, what conclusions would you draw about George's knowledge regarding diabetes and his subsequent ability to perform glucose monitoring and insulin injection?

22. In the interactions with the nurse, George Gonzalez makes a statement about how he has managed his diabetes previously. What does he say about his daily monitoring of glucose and administration of insulin before going to school?

21

Diabetes Care and Self-Management

Reading Assignments:
  Hockenberry: Wong's Essentials of Pediatric Nursing, 10th edition (Chapters 14, 19, and 28)
  Hockenberry: Wong's Nursing Care of Infants and Children, 10th edition
          (Chapters 1, 15, 19, and 33)

Patient: George Gonzalez, Room 301

Objectives:

1. Describe the significance of glucose monitoring, diet, and exercise in the management of the child with type 1 diabetes mellitus (DM).
2. Discuss the impact of a chronic illness on the preadolescent child and family.
3. Identify potential complications of type 1 DM in relation to poor glycemic control.
4. Identify specific learning needs of the preadolescent with a chronic illness.

Exercise 1

Virtual Hospital Activity

55 minutes

- Sign in to work at Pacific View Regional Hospital for Period of Care 2. (*Note:* If you are already in the virtual hospital from a previous exercise, click on **Leave the Floor** and then on **Restart the Program** to get to the sign-in window.)
- From the Patient List, select George Gonzalez (Room 301).
- Click on **Go to Nurses' Station**.
- Click on **Chart** and then on **301** for George Gonzalez's record.
- Click on and review the **Nurse's Notes** and **Physician's Notes**.
- Click on **Return to Nurses' Station** and then on **301** to go to George Gonzalez's room.
- Click on **Patient Care** and then on **Nurse-Client Interactions**.

151

- Select and view the video titled **1115: Teaching—Disease Process**. (*Note:* Check the virtual clock to see whether enough time has elapsed. You can use the fast-forward feature to advance the time by 2-minute intervals if the video is not yet available. Then click again on **Patient Care** and **Nurse-Client Interactions** to refresh the screen.)
- Now view the video titled **1130: Teaching—Managing Symptoms**.

1. What does George Gonzalez's mother say about his diabetes management?

2. What does George Gonzalez's mother tell the nurse about recognizing George's need for insulin?

3. The nurse discusses with the mother signs indicating George Gonzalez may need insulin. What are the signs of hyperglycemia in a child George's age?

4. During these two video interactions, what is the nurse evaluating in regard to knowledge of diabetes management?

5. What does George Gonzalez tell the nurse about the signs of hypoglycemia? What does he think he should do if he feels hypoglycemic?

- To answer the following two questions, you may need to return to Period of Care 1 and view the nurse's interactions with George Gonzalez and his mother. If you need help changing periods of care, see **A Quick Tour** in this workbook.

6. Briefly summarize your impressions regarding the following issues.

   a. George Gonzalez's previous management of diabetes in relation to glucose monitoring and insulin administration:

   b. George Gonzalez's mother's knowledge about the importance of daily diabetes management:

7. Briefly summarize the main teaching points the nurse has covered up to this point with George Gonzalez and his mother regarding diabetes management.

8. What could the nurse emphasize with George Gonzalez and his mother about diabetes management to help control his blood glucose and prevent further hospitalizations?

- Click on **Chart** and then on **301**.
- Review the **History and Physical** and the **Nursing Admission**.
- Next, click on **Consultations** and review the Psychiatric Consult.

9. According to the History and Physical, George Gonzalez has been hospitalized for problems with diabetes. What specific problems has he had with diabetes management in the last 4 months?

10. List two patient problems for George Gonzalez based on what you have learned from his chart and the nurse-client video interactions.

11. Briefly describe George Gonzalez's family situation (parents, siblings, primary care provider).

12. There are insights to George Gonzalez's previous diabetes management patterns found in the Nursing Admission, History and Physical, and Psychiatric Consult in the chart. List four factors that have contributed to George's noncompliance with his diabetes regimen in the last 4 months.

13. What involvement is expected of George Gonzalez's family, given his age and developmental stage?

14. George Gonzalez has had diabetes for 4 years. Briefly describe the effect of a chronic illness such as diabetes on a preadolescent and his family.

Exercise 2

Virtual Hospital Activity

20 minutes

- Sign in to work at Pacific View Regional Hospital for Period of Care 3. (*Note:* If you are already in the virtual hospital from a previous exercise, click on **Leave the Floor** and then on **Restart the Program** to get to the sign-in window.)
- From the Patient List, select George Gonzalez (Room 301).
- Click on **Go to Nurses' Station**.
- Click on **Chart** and then on **301** for George Gonzalez's record.
- Click on **Consultations** and review the Nutrition Consult.
- Click on **Return to Nurses' Station**.
- Click on **301** to go to George Gonzalez's room.
- Inside his room, click on **Patient Care** and then on **Nurse-Client Interactions**.
- Select and view the video titled **1500: Teaching—Diabetic Diet**. (*Note:* Check the virtual clock to see whether enough time has elapsed. You can use the fast-forward feature to advance the time by 2-minute intervals if the video is not yet available. Then click again on **Patient Care** and **Nurse-Client Interactions** to refresh the screen.)

1. What is George Gonzalez's recommended dietary intake?

2. What does the nurse discuss with George Gonzalez in regard to his food intake?

3. What has been George Gonzalez's pattern of eating in the last several months?

4. Describe the relationship of food intake to insulin injections in a child with type 1 DM.

5. How does carbohydrate counting give more flexibility in making food choices and administering insulin in children with type 1 DM?

- Click on **Patient Care** and then on **Nurse-Client Interactions**.
- Select and view the video titled **1535: Teaching—Effects of Exercise**. (*Note:* Check the virtual clock to see whether enough time has elapsed. You can use the fast-forward feature to advance the time by 2-minute intervals if the video is not yet available. Then click again on **Patient Care** and **Nurse-Client Interactions** to refresh the screen.)

6. What activity does George Gonzalez say he really likes?

7. Why is exercise an important part of the management of type 1 diabetes?

8. Identify important items in the following areas that the nurse should discuss with George Gonzalez in relation to diabetes management and exercise.

   a. Glucose monitoring

   b. Carbohydrate intake

c. When not to exercise

d. Signs of activity intolerance

9. What specific intervention does George Gonzalez promise to get involved in following discharge that is aimed at helping him manage his diabetes effectively? (*Hint:* If necessary, return to his chart and review the **Consultations**.)

Notes:

Notes:

Notes:

Notes:

Notes:

Notes:

Notes:

Notes: